48

Delux

Gill Paul

First published in 2008 by
Collins, an imprint of HarperCollins Publishers Ltd.
77-85 Fulham Palace Road, London, W6 8JB

www.collins.co.uk

Collins is a registered trademark of HarperCollins Publishers Ltd.

Created by: SP Creative Design
Editor: Heather Thomas: Designer: Rolando Ugolini

A catalogue record for this book is available from the British Library.

ISBN 978-0-00-726658-6

Collins uses papers that are natural, renewable and recyclable products made
from wood grown in sustainable forests. The manufacturing processes
conform to the environmental regulations of the country of origin.

Printed and bound in Italy by Amadeus

Mixed Sources
Product group from well-managed
forests and other controlled sources
www.fsc.org Cert no. SW-COC-1806
© 1996 Forest Stewardship Council

FSC

FSC is a non-profit international organisation established to promote the
responsible management of the world's forests. Products carrying the FSC
label are independently certified to assure consumers that they come
from forests that are managed to meet the social, economic and
ecological needs of present and future generations.

Find out more about HarperCollins and the environment at
www.harpercollins.co.uk/green

This is a general reference book and although care has been taken to
ensure the information is as up-to-date and accurate as possible, it is no
substitute for professional advice based on your personal circumstances.
Consult your doctor before making any major changes to your diet.

CONTENTS

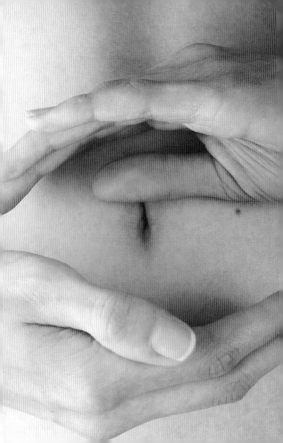

PART 1

HOW TOXIC ARE YOU?

The human body is very sophisticated, performing a huge range of essential functions simultaneously right round the clock. Filtering out and eliminating any materials that could cause the body harm is crucial. Over the centuries, as technology has developed, the toxins to which we are exposed have changed and the body has adapted to deal with new ones, but in the last 60 years there has been a big increase in the number of chemicals in our air, water, food and everyday surroundings. Are we still coping or are we heading for overload?

YOUR BODY'S DEFENCES

The liver, kidneys, spleen, digestive system, respiratory system, lymphatic system and skin all work together to try and keep potentially harmful substances (toxins) out of our bodies, or to neutralize them if they do get in. So how well are your body's defences working?

WHAT IS A TOXIN?

Toxins are substances that can harm us when they are ingested into the body. If asked to name some toxins, most people would mention alcohol, tobacco and caffeine first, and they would be right in so far as these are all substances that can cause significant harm to the body. They are deliberately ingested toxins, but there are many more we don't consume deliberately and may not even be aware of.

Quit smoking

Cigarettes contain up to 600 additives and when these are set on fire, the smoke contains over 4,000 chemicals, of which over 50 are known to be cancer-forming. They include radioactive Polonium-210, found in tobacco that is grown in fields which are fertilized with phosphates, and even Zyklon B, a gas that was used by the Nazis for mass extermination in the death camps.

A good cry

Our eyes have their own defence system to prevent toxins getting in. Eyelashes sweep away larger particles, while tears contain an enzyme called lysozyme, which can destroy bacteria, and the liquid washes away micro-organisms.

Toxins in our environment

Some toxins are in the air we breathe, the water we drink and the foods, even seemingly healthy ones, that we eat. For example, when you eat a strawberry that has been sprayed with pesticide to kill any bugs in the strawberry patch, you ingest the pesticide along with the vitamin C and antioxidants of the fruit.

When you stand on a city street and breathe in, your lungs have to cope with a cocktail of exhaust fumes and other gases, among which is the oxygen we need to stay alive. When you drink mineral water, you could be consuming traces of antimony, a poison that has been found in plastic bottles, alongside the water that you need for survival.

Therefore, in our high-tech, modern society, we are surrounded by toxins at every turn, no matter how hard we try to be healthy. Fortunately, however, our bodies have ways of dealing with most of the substances they come into contact with and, as we shall see, there are positive things you can do to minimize their effect.

PREVENTION IS THE BEST DEFENCE

To get into the body, toxins have to be inhaled, eaten or absorbed through the skin. The first-line defences try to prevent entry in the first place, but, if they fail, there are second and third lines in waiting.

Respiratory system

When you breathe in through your nose, tiny hairs – cilia – filter out particles of dust and soot, which will be expelled the next time you sneeze or blow your nose. The mucous membranes lining the mouth and nose contain a chemical called lactoferrin, which destroys bacteria, and saliva also has antibacterial ingredients. As air travels down the respiratory tract, more cilia and mucous membranes remove unwanted particles and phlegm is produced to ferry them upwards, triggering sensors that induce us to cough.

In the lungs, the air enters sacs known as alveoli, where the white blood cells identify dust or potential toxins and they release the appropriate toxin-killing cells. At least, this is the case in normal, healthy adults; those with asthma or other lung problems don't fight toxins quite so successfully.

Digestive system

When you eat or drink something, the antibacterial compounds in the mouth work on it first, and then

Your bowel movements

Ideally, food remains should pass through the digestive system within 24 hours. However, most of us retain waste products in our colon for between two and seven days – or even longer – meaning that toxic substances have a good chance of being reabsorbed into the bloodstream again.

stomach acid kills off a lot of potentially dangerous toxins before they get further down the intestine.

Once in the intestine, beneficial bacteria ('friendly' in the TV ads) help to defend the system from poisons, while microscopic villi absorb nutrients into the blood stream. The small intestine, which is 6m (20ft) in length, filters out any larger molecules and undigested foods and carries them down to be excreted when you have a bowel movement. Smaller molecules that are absorbed are carried in the first instance to the liver.

Liver and gall bladder

The liver is a multi-tasking organ which produces and processes hundreds of chemicals every day. When blood arrives from the small intestine, the liver secretes enzymes that process vital nutrients into a form in which they can be used by the cells of the body. It stores excess glucose (sugar) as glycogen and produces cholesterol, a substance that helps the blood to carry fats around the body. It also clears the blood of drugs and poisons, breaking them down to neutralize them or turning them into a form in which they can be secreted as bile fluid. Bile is transported from the liver to the gall bladder, and when you next eat something containing fat, the bile is excreted into the small intestine to help the digestive process and, if the system is functioning effectively, the bile will then pass from your body in faeces.

Kidneys

The kidneys filter about 200 litres of blood every day, sifting out waste products and excess water. A series of tiny tubes called nephrons are the filtering units. Most of us make about 2 litres (3 1/2 pints) of urine a day from substances that are no longer needed by the body.

Spleen

Another of the body's filtering systems, the spleen removes worn-out red blood cells from circulation and recycles them into iron to build the blood. It also gets rid of any unhealthy bacteria, so it can stop you going down with colds or flu when it is functioning efficiently.

Lymphatic system

White blood cells (the ones that fight disease) are stored in lymph nodes situated under your arms, in your neck, around your spine and in your groin. You may be able to feel that your lymph nodes are swollen when you are fighting off an infection. A watery fluid

Exercise

The lymphatic system does not have a pump – in the way that the blood circulates due to the action of the heart – so it can be sluggish if you don't get much exercise.

called lymph is circulated round the body, mainly by the action of your muscles. In the cells, lymph is responsible for filtering out the waste products of cellular reactions and other toxins that have got into the tissues. It also carries white blood cells to sites of infection, where they adhere to and break down micro-organisms and debris that they recognize as foreign.

Skin

The average adult has 1.6 square metres (3 square yards) of skin forming a barrier between the body's internal organs and the outside world. Bacteria and micro-organisms cannot pass through unbroken skin, and are prevented from multiplying by the action of oily sebum secreted by the sebaceous glands at the root of hair follicles. Sweat also contains antibacterial lactoferrin.

However, if the skin is broken, by a cut or graze, bacteria and micro-organisms can get into the body and the immune system has to send white blood cells to kill them. Chemicals are released that cause the area to become red, hot and inflamed as blood vessels widen to speed white blood cells to the site.

Some chemicals can pass through unbroken skin, but only very slowly. Thus the nicotine in nicotine patches makes its way into the bloodstream, as do certain toxic chemicals, such as insecticides and solvents.

The skin is also an organ for the secretion of waste products. As you heat up and perspire, you release toxins from the fatty tissues. The more you sweat, the more you release, which is why saunas can be an effective part of a general detox programme.

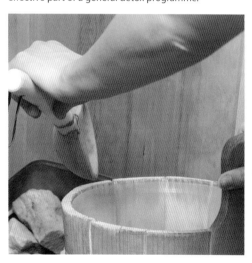

Hormone trouble

Toxins in the blood disturb the action of our hormones, leading to problems, such as acne in teenagers, PMS (premenstrual syndrome), heavy periods and menopausal symptoms in women, and hair loss in men. Conventional medical treatments may involve taking synthetic hormones, such as the Pill or HRT (hormone replacement therapy), adding another layer of hormones for the liver to deal with.

WASTE DISPOSAL SYSTEM OVERLOAD

In 1999 and 2000, the American Centers for Disease Control and Prevention tested 2,500 people for 116 different toxic chemicals and found that in every case, they were storing several. *The Sunday Times* published similar findings in the UK in 2004. In all instances, they measured scary levels of toxic chemicals, including: polychlorinated biphenyls (PCBs), banned since the 1970s; DDT, a pesticide banned in the UK and US; dioxins; and heavy metals, including lead, cadmium, mercury and aluminium.

Did you know?

- More than 80,000 different industrial chemicals are now licensed for use.
- The average British adult is thought to consume 5kg (11lb) of food additives a year, and 4.5 litres (8 pints) of pesticides on their fruit and vegetables.

Autism

In his 2006 book *Autism, Brain and Environment*, Richard Lathe suggests that the huge increase in cases of autism in recent years could be due to an increase in environmental toxins, including pesticides, lead, PCBs and mercury. He suggests that many cases are caused by a genetic weakness that means the system can't deal adequately with such toxins, leading to brain damage that causes the psychological problems connected with the syndrome.

• Up to 25 per cent of the US population suffer from heavy metal poisoning from lead, cadmium, mercury and aluminium. Heavy metal toxicity is linked to several diseases, including Alzheimer's and Parkinson's.
• In 1940, it took four months to raise a chicken from when it hatched until it weighed around 2kg (4lb) and was ready to eat. In 1990, it took just six weeks because the additives in chicken food have been designed to fatten them up quickly. These same additives can make it harder for us to lose weight when we ingest them through eating chicken. Battery-farm-reared chickens also contain antibiotics, which are given routinely to prevent disease in their over-crowded conditions.
• More and more fish caught around the world contain such high levels of mercury that governments are advising pregnant women not to eat the larger fish, such as tuna, which have the highest concentrations. One study found that women who ate more than two

Heavy metals

Arsenic, cadmium, lead and mercury can't be broken down in the body, so they accumulate and cause damage at even low levels. They are found in many common substances:

• Arsenic can be ingested from food and water that has been contaminated, or breathing smoke from burning wood treated with copper-chromated arsenic.

• Cadmium can be found in water and foods that come from the water, especially shellfish.

• Lead is found in pipes, paints and solder in old houses.

• Mercury is found in dental fillings, vaccinations, and contaminated fish and shellfish.

servings of fish per week had a higher risk of having a child with autism; 57 per cent of mothers of children with attention deficit disorder were found to have high levels of mercury in their bodies.

• Fluoride, added to tap water in many areas to protect the teeth, can build up in the soil, in plants and in our bones. It can cause osteoporosis, and some studies link it to hypothyroidism, which affects 10–25 per cent of the British population. Fluoride can make it harder for the immune system to distinguish foreign substances from the body's own tissue, leading to skin rashes and intestinal disorders, while several studies link fluoride with genetic disorders.

• Chemicals that mimic the effects of oestrogen in the body are present in many household cleaning products,

Food additives

Long lists of E numbers in the ingredients of a foodstuff should make you wary. Some additives have protective or preservative functions, but others are just used to colour foods or enhance flavours. The following have all been associated with the side effects noted:

• Tartrazine (E102) – may suppress the immune system and can cause hyperactivity in children, allergies, asthma, migraines, even cancer.

• Sunset yellow (E110) – can be particularly dangerous for asthmatics and for anyone who is sensitive to aspirin.

• Amaranth (E123) – may suppress the immune system and has been banned in the US since 1976.

• Erythrosine (E127) – mimics the action of oestrogen in the body and can be carcinogenic.

• Sodium benzoate (E211) – linked to behaviour problems in children.

• Calcium propionate (E282) – linked to attention deficit and sleep problems in children.

• Butylated hydroxyanisole (BTGA – E320) – linked to attention deficit, irritability and asthma; banned in Japan.

• Monosodium glutamate (E621) – can cause headaches, giddiness, nausea, muscle pains, heart palpitations, irritability, attention problems.

• Ribonucleotides (E635) – linked to allergies and behaviour problems in children.

• Aspartame (E951) – linked to headaches, mood swings, fatigue and allergies.

including some washing-up liquids and fabric softeners, cosmetics, such as lipstick and nail polish, hair dyes and many other substances. This is one cause of oestrogen dominance, a hormonal imbalance that affects men and women throughout the Western world.

● Formaldehyde, found in new carpets and processed wood furniture among other things, can irritate the eyes, nose and throat at just low levels.

● A ready-washed bag of salad contains chlorine levels 20 times higher than in most swimming pools. Chlorine was one of the poisonous gases used in World War I.

● Volatile organic compounds (VOCs) are found in aerosol sprays, dry-cleaned clothes, paint, paint strippers and petrol – there are more than 200 VOCs in common UK household products. Some studies indicate that VOCs may damage the nervous and immune systems and that they have been linked to brain tumours, childhood leukaemia and childhood asthma.

● Phthalates, used to make all sorts of household goods from toys to wallpaper, have been linked to liver and thyroid damage, cancer, low sperm counts in men, miscarriages in women, and birth defects in babies.

Note: This list could stretch over several pages – in fact, there are many entire books about the huge quantities of brand-new toxins that are being created by industry, and plenty of evidence that these toxins are making their way through our bodies' defence systems to be stored in the fatty tissue, blood and bones.

WHAT TOXINS DO TO US

We have looked at how the body's waste disposal systems work in 'normal' circumstances, but what can go wrong if they become overloaded with more toxins than they can deal with, or with new ones that they do not recognize?

UNDERFUNCTIONING LUNGS

When they are assaulted daily by air pollutants, the cilia and the mucous membranes in the respiratory system become less effective. The alveoli get furred up with tarry substances, meaning that less of the surface area across which oxygen is absorbed to the blood is available. Less oxygen in the system makes us get tired more easily, so our muscles ache more readily on exertion. Overall, we feel more sluggish.

Stress

When we are stressed, our heartbeat rises, more sugar is released into the bloodstream and the hormones cortisol and adrenaline are released, both of which promote fat storage in the abdomen. People who are frequently stressed are prone to getting into a pattern of compulsive eating, drinking or smoking. Stress is a toxic emotion all round but it can be combated.

Asthma

The incidence of asthma has been rising steadily since 1970. It is now four times higher in adults and six times higher in children than it was back then. According to Asthma UK, environmental pollution may play a part in causing it and certainly makes symptoms worse. The weight of medical evidence suggests that active or passive exposure to cigarette smoke in the early years of life increases the risk of developing asthma.

Hay fever

About 15 per cent of the population in industrialized countries now suffer from hay fever. It has a much higher prevalence in urban areas than rural settings, and increases are particularly striking in areas of high pollution. Like asthma, it is an allergic disease, but it seems that our atmosphere is making us much more prone to these conditions, and, once you have a respiratory disease like this, it becomes harder for your lungs to fight off other toxins.

LEAKY GUT

Only a few substances are absorbed directly through the stomach, and these include alcohol, aspirin, cigarette smoke and certain other noxious chemicals. If the stomach lining has been assaulted too often in this way, it can become 'leaky'. Further down in the intestine, the same thing can happen due to our intake

Coeliac disease

This is a hypersensitivity to gluten, a protein found in rye, wheat and certain other cereals. The damage it causes to the gut can prevent absorption of other foods, leading to vitamin and mineral deficiencies, weight loss, abdominal pain, tiredness and a host of other unpleasant symptoms. Once the sensitivity develops, it is permanent, and the only thing you can do is to avoid gluten for the rest of your life.

of antibiotics, caffeine, chemicals in processed foods, prescription corticosteroids, or even just a diet that is full of highly refined carbohydrates, such as sweets, cakes, biscuits, white bread and pizza.

Once you have a 'leaky gut', the spaces between cell walls are larger and allow larger molecules of bacteria, waste matter and undigested food into the bloodstream. Your immune system views these substances as 'alien' and acts to eliminate them. Antibodies are made against these proteins derived from previously harmless foods, and these antibodies can trigger an inflammatory reaction next time the corresponding food is eaten.

Food allergies

If you have a food allergy, you will get an immediate and usually severe reaction, but intolerances may have less clear-cut symptoms, manifesting in different parts of the body over the longer term. They are generally not life-threatening but can make you feel unwell. To diagnose an intolerance, avoid the food you suspect for a period of months and see if the symptoms clear up.

CLOGGED-UP COLON

A common symptom of toxin overload and a diet that is dependent on processed foods is a clogged-up colon. Normally the colon produces just enough mucus to move faeces along, but when toxins, drugs or stress irritate it, it produces excess mucus which can bind with starchy waste materials to make hardened faeces. These become impacted in pockets in the colon, so the villi cannot absorb nutrients efficiently and the gap through which waste has to pass becomes narrower.

The build-up becomes a breeding ground for bacteria and parasites (such as tapeworms and flukes), and you become constipated. In some people, a hard mass can actually be felt in the lower abdomen. They will probably suffer from flatulence, as the trapped food ferments, giving off gases and sulphur-containing compounds which give that characteristic smell.

Another problem is that the longer waste material sits around without being eliminated, the more chance there is that the toxins in it will be reabsorbed by the body. Some people even have faecal material in their colons that has been there for several years!

Stools test

You can check your stools, according to the following list, to see how healthy your gut really is. When you go to the toilet, look before you flush!

• Eat some sweetcorn to test how quickly food is moving through your gut. You should be able to spot undigested husks when they come out the other end. This should take 24 hours or less.

• Do your stools float? This is good, but if they are so buoyant that you have trouble flushing them away, then your liver is out of balance.

• How do they smell? Very smelly stools are a sign that your colon is clogged up and waste products are stagnating in there.

• How many wipes does it take to clean your bottom? More than three wipes and you are producing too much mucus, which means that your colon is irritated. (This is also the case if you leave skid marks on the loo.)

• If you observe that your stools are tiny, hard pellets, then your liver is congested.

• Stools should be a walnut colour. If yours are very light-coloured, it means that you are having trouble digesting fatty foods.

• Thin, shreddy stools are another sign of a clogged-up colon.

• Loose stools could be caused by a bug, or they could be a sign that your spleen is exhausted.

FATTY LIVER

Toxic compounds, such as alcohol, solvents, heavy metals, paracetamol, penicillin and hormones, are processed by the liver in two stages. They are changed into an intermediate form, which is even more toxic, before they can bind to an amino acid or nutrient to help their elimination in bile. If the process is interrupted, because the liver has so many other substances to deal with, the intermediate toxic compounds can circulate in the blood, causing all kinds of damage.

If the liver is not getting the substances it needs to make bile, you will have trouble digesting food, particularly fatty foods. Bile can become congested with filtered elements and will get backed up in the bile ducts. In this case, you won't be able to metabolize fats and you will gain weight, and the toxins and their by-products will remain in your circulation.

Alcohol

This is broken down by the liver to acetaldehyde, a toxic compound that leaches vitamins B and C and causes the kidneys to excrete more fluid, along with zinc, magnesium and potassium. The classic hangover symptoms are caused by dehydration, but this can be fixed by drinking lots of water to rehydrate. On a more sinister note, the free radicals formed by acetaldehyde will be attacking cells and causing them to degenerate.

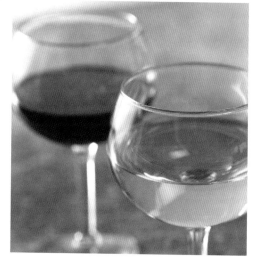

Drinking too much?

More than one in five men and almost one in 10 women binge drink every week, consuming more than eight units of alcohol a day for men and more than six for women. Excessive alcohol intake is the most common cause of sudden fits in young men. A woman's risk of getting breast cancer rises by six per cent for each extra drink she has on a daily basis, and she's at more risk of brain damage than men.

A liver that has to deal with excess toxins, particularly alcohol, will begin to form fatty deposits inside its cells. Fatty liver is now recognized as the most common cause of abnormal liver function tests in the West, with around 20 per cent of the UK population suffering from it. Long-term exposure to acetaldehyde causes scarring of the liver tissue leading to cirrhosis. There has been a sharp rise in liver cirrhosis deaths in the UK over the last 20 years, more than doubling for people in Scotland and increasing by two-thirds for men in England.

Regenerating the liver

However, if you stop the damage before it reaches the cirrhosis stage, the liver can break up its fatty tissues and regenerate itself remarkably well. Even if you just give up drinking for a week or a month, you give your liver a chance to catch up on the backlog; all drinkers, even moderate ones, should do this from time to time.

KIDNEY STONES

Stones form in the kidneys when urine stays too long in the system, so drinking plenty of liquid is essential to keep them eliminating waste efficiently. Urine should be a pale straw colour and you should produce at least 2 litres (3½ pints) per day, on around five to six trips to the lavatory. Any darker than this, and any less volume, and you are not drinking enough water, so toxins are sitting around longer than need be inside you.

It's in the eyes

Look at your eyes to see how well your liver is functioning. Are the whites white or a dull cream or yellowy colour? Do you have dark shadows under your eyes? Both are signs of a liver that is struggling to eliminate toxins.

WEIGHT PROBLEMS

If your digestive system and liver are not functioning effectively, it is difficult to control your weight. A toxic liver can't metabolize fat and cholesterol and dumps them back in the bloodstream. Many toxins are stored in body fat, and the more fat you have, the more waste you collect. Conversely, the more toxins in your system, the fatter you are likely to be.

According to the World Health Organization, 76 per cent of British men between 30 and 69 years are overweight, compared with 65 per cent 10 years ago; 69 per cent of women are overweight compared with 55 per cent in 1995. One in five men and women are categorized as clinically obese. As a nation, we are getting fatter and fatter, making us much more at risk of life-threatening diseases, such as diabetes, heart disease and cancers. Our fat stores, particularly abdominal fat, become metabolically active. A waist measurement of more than 90cm (36in) in men (80cm (32in) in women) is associated with increased risk of metabolic complications.

Waist-to-hip ratio

This is now a recognized clinical method of evaluating abdominal fat. The waist is measured at the narrowest point, whereas the hips are measured at the widest point, and then the waist measurement divided by the hip measurement gives the waist-to-hip ratio. If higher than 1.0 for men and 0.85 for women, you have too much abdominal fat and are putting your health at risk.

Cellulite

This is the orange-peel dimply flesh that some women get on their hips and thighs. Men get it too, but they have more muscle tissue to disguise it. It is caused by sluggish circulation: lymph fluid and toxins accumulate between connective tissues. Hormone supplements, such as the Pill or HRT, can contribute to the build up of cellulite, as can such factors as stress, a sedentary lifestyle, lack of exercise and binge eating.

Cancer link

The American Cancer Society produced a study in 2003 which found that the more overweight a person is, the higher their chance of developing many types of cancer. Excess weight was a factor in 20 per cent of cancer deaths in women and 14 per cent in men. Obese women are two to four times more likely to get endometrial and kidney cancer, twice as likely to get pancreatic cancer and 46 per cent more likely to get colon cancer.

SKIN PROBLEMS

The skin is a mirror that shows not only how well your elimination organs are working, but also the level of toxins in your body and whether you lack vitamins and minerals in your diet. If your skin is very reactive, prone to spots, blotches, rashes, eczema or psoriasis, you probably need to clean out. Toxicity will also make you look more tired and wrinkly, and your skin tone will be yellowy or greyish rather than clear and glowing.

COMPROMISED IMMUNITY

When a person is exposed to a new toxin they have not encountered before, they respond with physiological shock. Blood flow to the area is decreased while the body works out how to deal with the toxin and adapts. When the system is overloaded with new toxins, the adaptation

Infertility

According to a study in *The Lancet,* average sperm count in British men fell from 113 million per millilitre in 1940 to 66 million in 1990. Between eight and twelve per cent are now functionally sterile, with a sperm count of less than 20 million per millilitre. Women with repeated miscarriages typically have partners with low sperm counts. Poor diet plus excessive alcohol and caffeine are the main cause; as are oestrogens in water, food and the environment.

Tongue diagnosis

Practitioners of Traditional Chinese Medicine (TCM) will check your tongue when making a diagnosis, because it is a good indicator of general health. A healthy tongue should be pale red with a thin white film, and smooth and moist. Is yours like this, or do you recognize the following?

- A thick yellow coating: bowels aren't working efficiently.
- A thick white coating on the tongue: too much mucus in the system and not enough beneficial bacteria in the gut.
- A crack down the middle of the tongue: a weak stomach. If you have this, you are probably prone to bloating.
- Watch out for cracks, teeth marks and red patches on the tongue. Depending on location, they indicate that an organ is underfunctioning. The right side of the tongue shows the performance of the gall bladder, the left side is the liver, the middle is the stomach and spleen, while the back of the tongue mirrors the kidneys, intestine, bladder and womb.

process is less successful and a range of symptoms can set in, including allergies, psoriasis, arthritis and asthma, plus hormone fluctuations and mental problems.

While your body is struggling with a range of toxins, the immune system can become compromised, making you more prone to picking up opportunistic infections, such as colds, flu and herpes cold sores. If you feel you get more than your fair share of bugs, it might be worth thinking about taking steps to reduce your toxic load.

DO YOU NEED TO DETOX?

There are many, many more effects of toxins on the body and not enough space to list them all here. If you are still unsure about whether you have a toxic overload which is dragging down your general physical and mental functioning, then answer the questions in the box below and add up the number of ticks.

Self assessment

If you have ticked even just one of the questions below in the self assessment questionnaire, then the chances

Examine yourself

☐ Have you taken more than two or three doses of antibiotics in your life?

☐ Do you often feel sleepy after eating a meal?

☐ Do you ever get cravings for specific foods?

☐ Are you gassy? Do you burp, fart or get bloated after eating fatty foods?

☐ Do you often get a bitter taste in your mouth?

☐ Do you have bad breath or smelly body odour? (Ask a close friend!)

☐ Do you suffer from joint stiffness/muscle weakness?

☐ Do you often feel fatigued for no reason?

☐ Do you frequently wake between 1am and 3am and are not sure why?

☐ Do you have trouble sleeping?

are that you have a toxic burden which is affecting your health. Basically, even people who live on remote islands cannot avoid pollutants altogether, although some are more reactive than others.

Gentle is best

There is some controversy in the medical profession about the notion of 'detoxification', as some of the extreme methods can do more harm than good, but in the next chapter, we will take a look at how a gentle detox programme could help you to start to shift some of your toxins and in the process make you feel much, much better.

☐ Do you find it hard to concentrate?

☐ Are you worried about your memory?

☐ Do you get drunk more easily than your friends?

☐ Are you depressed for no obvious reason?

☐ Do you get more colds than your contemporaries?

☐ Do you often get a stuffy, blocked-up nose?

For women

☐ Have you tried unsuccessfully to get pregnant?

☐ Do you suffer from PMS or pronounced menopausal symptoms, such as hot flushes?

For men

☐ Do you have problems getting and maintaining an erection?

☐ Has your partner had trouble conceiving a baby?

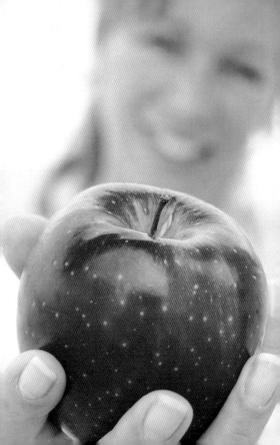

PART 2

How detoxing works

Detoxing should never be entered into suddenly, without preparation or after a period of excess. Indeed, many medical experts advise against it altogether because of the harm it can do if your body is not ready to deal with the mass release of its stored toxins. However, follow the gentle, step-by-step approach in this chapter and you can begin to cleanse your system. Be aware that you won't get rid of years of ingested toxins with just 48 hours of good behaviour. Get ready for the long haul if you are serious about improving your health.

BODY SHOCK

If you have never tried detoxing before, start at the beginning of this chapter and then work your way through slowly. Even if you have detoxed in the past and don't have any serious bad habits, it is still worth refreshing yourself on what to do.

CUT OUT BAD HABITS

Some detox programmes will suggest cutting down overnight to a diet of raw vegetable juices plus the recommended vitamin and herbal supplements. They require you to go cold turkey on caffeine, alcohol, wheat, dairy foods, salt, sugar, processed foods and many other toxin-laden or difficult-to-digest substances. However, it's extreme plans like these that have given detoxification a bad name in certain medical circles, because they would make you feel very ill if you sustained them over a long period.

A lifetime's worth of pesticide residues, drugs and other poisons stored in the fat cells is suddenly broken down and released into the bloodstream, causing all kinds of unpleasant symptoms. These can seriously compromise your immune and nervous systems and interfere with the action of your thyroid gland, and you would have been much better off staying as you were.

A balanced regime

Another criticism that the medical establishment fires at detox diets is that they are lacking in protein and essential nutrients needed by the liver to metabolize food. You will learn how to select detox foods and drinks to keep your diet balanced. The first step is to cut out bad habits, such as smoking, excessive alcohol or caffeine, use of street drugs or over-the-counter medication.

Quick-fix detox diets

Like crash diets, these are not successful methods of losing weight, because when your body is deprived of food it goes into starvation mode and will retain all the calories it can to supply energy. When you start eating normally again, your metabolism will still be programmed to retain calories and so you could put on weight very rapidly.

WARNING: Don't stop taking any prescription medication without discussing it with your doctor.

SMOKING

If you are ready to quit, there are many organizations, books, tapes, herbal remedies and complementary therapies to help you (see page 182). Oat straw, a source of B vitamins which is available from health food shops, can help reduce the cravings and irritability that are experienced by many people giving up smoking.

ALCOHOL ABUSE

If you regularly consume more than two units of alcohol a day (for women) or three (for men), or if you drink more than six units in one session, you're putting your health at serious risk. One in three heavy drinkers will die in middle age because of drinking, even though they might not consider themselves to be 'alcoholics'.

Seeking help

Cut out alcohol completely at least seven days before you go on a detox. Your liver will start to recover straight away. If you can't do this, you may need to seek help. Talk to your GP or call Alcoholics Anonymous (see page 182). A Chinese remedy called kudzu, which is available from alternative chemists or from Traditional Chinese Medicine (TCM) centres, can be useful for combating cravings when you give up alcohol. Take 150mg three times a day, and drink lots of water.

How much is a unit?

A unit depends on the strength of the alcoholic drink. To work out how many units there are in, say, a bottle or can, multiply the percentage of alcohol by the volume of liquid and divide the answer by 100 if the volume is in centilitres (1,000 if in millilitres). Thus a 75cl bottle of wine with an alcohol content of 12 would be:

12 x 75 ÷ 100 = 9 units of alcohol per bottle.

Do you get enough sleep?

Inadequate sleep lowers our immune response. Several studies have shown that missing even a few hours a night on a regular basis can decrease the number of 'natural killer cells', which are responsible for fighting off bacteria and viruses. People who suffer from insomnia may find they succumb to colds and other illnesses more frequently than their partners who sleep through the night.

OVER-THE-COUNTER DRUGS

An estimated 30,000 people in the UK are addicted to over-the-counter (OTC) medications, with painkillers at the top of the list and cough medicines second. There are many side effects of this kind of dependency. One study found that regular use of ibuprofen doubles the risk of suffering a heart attack and increases the risk of stroke. Long-term misuse of painkillers can lead to physical and psychological dependency, constipation, headaches, nausea, liver dysfunction, gastrointestinal disorders, depression, mood swings, chronic lethargy and restless limbs. The warnings on packets state that if you take these drugs for longer than three days you should see your doctor to get treatment for the underlying illnesses that cause the symptoms. Talk to a herbalist, homeopath or naturopath if you want to investigate a holistic path to feeling well enough that you no longer need OTC drugs.

Are you a sugar addict?

Sweet foods cause blood sugar peaks and troughs which give you mood swings and energy dips as well as affecting the performance of your liver, pancreas and spleen. You can substitute sugar with natural sweeteners, such as honey or fructose, and cut right back on the quantities.

CAFFEINE WITHDRAWAL

Caffeine is right up there with nicotine as one of the most addictive substances, and, just like nicotine, it can produce severe withdrawal symptoms when you cut it out. Remember that caffeine is found in fizzy drinks, chocolate and painkillers as well as in tea and coffee.

If you are used to having three or more doses of caffeine a day, you may experience withdrawal symptoms when you give it up, including headaches, irritability, an inability to concentrate, cravings, anxiety, fatigue, a runny nose and, possibly, nausea. Don't rush for some paracetamol, though, or you'll undo all the good work you've started. Use rosemary, peppermint or lavender aromatherapy oils applied to the temples, the pulse points behind the earlobes and the back of the neck to relieve headache and nausea. Chamomile tea is also good for the relief of mild to moderate headaches, and Bach flower essence Rescue Remedy can help (see page 135).

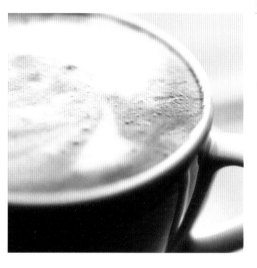

Are you a caffeine addict?

Caffeine makes the heart pump blood faster and has a diuretic effect. It can reduce fatigue and increase your concentration, but you quickly build up tolerance and need ever-greater doses to achieve the same effect. Strong coffee has around 200mg per cup, while strong tea has just 80mg, cola has 45–75mg and cocoa has just 10–15mg. Regular caffeine addicts can get withdrawal symptoms after just a few hours without their 'fix'.

Phasing out caffeine

If you have a real problem with caffeine withdrawal symptoms, you may need to take this slowly. Switch from coffee to green or black tea, which has caffeine but also contains bioflavonoids and catechin, which protects against heart disease and cancer and boosts the metabolism. When you are accustomed to drinking tea instead of coffee, cut back gradually by replacing a cup a day with herbal tea – there are lots of varieties you can try. Don't attempt to start a detox programme until you have sorted out your caffeine dependence or you will give your system too much to cope with.

ANTIOXIDANTS V. FREE RADICALS

Free radicals are unstable molecules that are created in the body as a result of some normal metabolic reactions. However, more are generated by smoking, drinking alcohol, environmental pollutants, taking antibiotics or paracetamol, or burning body fat on a weight-loss diet.

Free radicals have a negative electric charge and they try to neutralize this by colliding with other molecules, so they can pass on their spare electron in a process known as oxidation. Excess oxidation damages cell material and causes a number of degenerative problems and diseases, including atherosclerosis (furring and hardening of the arteries), heart disease, premature ageing and cancer.

Avoid grapefruit

Citrus fruits are all great sources of vitamin C, but avoid grapefruit when you are detoxing. It contains a substance that slows down the body's ability to process the toxins in alcohol, air pollution or prescription drugs. When scanning the menu in a cocktail bar, watch out for drinks containing grapefruit juice and alcohol and give them a wide berth.

Boost your antioxidants

The main defences against free radicals in the body are substances called antioxidants which can neutralize their negative electric charge before the damage is done. Antioxidants are nutrients taken in through your everyday diet and, as you prepare for a detox, it's crucial that you use this time to increase your antioxidant intake. By boosting your intake of foods containing the four major antioxidants, (carotenoids, Vitamins C and E and selenium) at the same time as cutting out alcohol and caffeine, your detox preparation will be boosted.

Carotenoids

These are found in yellow, orange, red and dark green fruits and vegetables, including carrots, tomatoes, spinach, sweetcorn, mangoes, peaches, watermelons and pumpkin. By reducing the oxidation of fats circulating in the blood, they diminish the risk of developing heart disease, cancers and cell damage, especially to the eyes.

Vitamin C

As well as being a powerful antioxidant, this vitamin prevents the conversion of nitrites (which are found in many processed meats and other pre-packaged foods) into carcinogenic nitrosamines. Vitamin C boosts the immune system, protecting us against a wide range of bacterial and viral diseases, cancers and heart disease. It also plays a role in helping to maintain sperm quality and prevent skin ageing. Rich sources of vitamin C include blueberries, kiwi fruits, blackberries, rosehips, oranges, red peppers, papaya, cantaloupe melon, broccoli and tomatoes.

Vitamin E

Food sources include avocado, eggs, nuts, seeds, whole grains, oily fish and broccoli, and should always be eaten raw where possible, because cooking destroys part of the vitamin E content. This crucial vitamin is the most important anti-ageing nutrient and it does seem to counteract some of the negative effects of pollution and heavy metals, while boosting the immune system and reducing the risk of heart disease and cancer.

Selenium

This valuable mineral binds to harmful toxins like mercury, arsenic and cadmium and strengthens the immune system's ability to destroy cancerous cells. You'll find it in Brazil nuts, fish, poultry, whole grains, mushrooms, onions, garlic, broccoli and cabbage.

BUMP UP YOUR FIBRE

Did you pass the stools test on page 22? You should have bowel movements at least once a day and pass well-formed, walnut-coloured, non-sticky stools that float on the surface of the water but flush away easily.

Are you getting enough fibre?

Many of the everyday foods we eat contain fibre, especially whole grain cereals, beans and pulses, vegetables and fruit. Look at the common foods listed below to see how you can boost your daily fibre intake:

1 bowl whole oat porridge (not instant)	8.5g
1/2 cup of kidney beans	7.9g
1/2 cup of chickpeas	7g
1 bowl of muesli	4.3g
1 medium apple	3.8g
1 handful of dried prunes	3.4g
1 medium pear	3.3g
1 large handful of sunflower seeds	3g
1 medium corn on the cob	2.5g
1 medium raw carrot	2.5g
1 slice of high-bran bread	2.4g
1 large handful of Brazil nuts	2g
1 portion of broccoli, boiled	1.4g
1 fist-sized portion of brown rice	0.6g

Recommended intake

In the UK, research studies show that most people get only about 12g of fibre a day from their diet, although the minimum recommended level is 18g and many experts say that 35g is optimum. Almost all of us would benefit from eating more fibre. When you're preparing for a detox it's essential that your bowels are moving food through efficiently, so you can get rid of all the toxins excreted from your cells instead of re-absorbing them. At least a week before a detox, start eating new sources of fibre until you can pass the stools test (see page 22). It's easy to do and requires only minimal dietary changes such as eating whole grain bread or cereal at breakfast or having fruit as snacks.

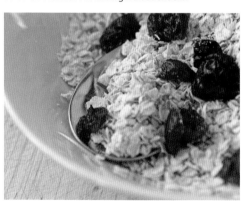

Irritable bowel syndrome

This condition causes intermittent abdominal pain, wind, nausea, bloating and alternating bouts of constipation and diahorrea. In 80 per cent of cases, IBS sufferers have an overgrowth of fungi, bacteria or parasites in their guts. Detoxing can help, under the supervision of a qualified therapist, and relaxation techniques can be beneficial.

Always add fibre gradually. If you add too much too quickly, you could experience uncomfortable bloating, wind and abdominal discomfort. Increase the amount of water you drink to eight 225ml (8fl oz) tumblers a day to wash down and bulk up the fibre in your diet.

CHOOSE A TIME

Choose a time to detox when you know you won't have important work commitments, as your concentration may be affected. A weekend may be best but avoid ones with social engagements as it will be hard to resist the pressure to join in, which may mean eating rich food and drinking alcohol. You may find that even on a 48-hour detox, you get more tired than usual, so ensure you get enough sleep. Don't choose a time when you have a sporting commitment, e.g. a tennis tournament or fun run – your performance will be affected and you could make yourself ill. The less obstacles you put in your way, the more successful you are likely to be.

DETOX GUIDELINES

If you have managed to give up alcohol and caffeine and bump up your antioxidant and fibre intake without experiencing more than mild side effects, then you are ready to try a proper detox, but before you start there are some general rules to consider.

BEFORE YOU START

Here are some guidelines to bear in mind before you start your 48-hour detox, which will help you to plan ahead and have a greater chance of success.

Is detoxing safe?

Ask your doctor if you have any ongoing health condition for which you are receiving treatment, e.g. diabetes, heart disease, hypoglycaemia, liver or kidney problems, thyroid problems, cancer or stomach ulcers. Do not detox if one of the following applies to you:

- If you are about to have, or just had, surgery.
- If you are on warfarin, blood pressure drugs, antidepressants or birth-control pills.
- If you are pregnant or breast-feeding.
- If you are under 18.
- If you have a mental illness, e.g. depression, anxiety, bipolar disorder, schizophrenia, eating disorder.

- Buy a wide range of the foods listed on the detox shopping list (see page 71).
- Decide which herbs and supplements you want to take (see pages 122) and buy them either by mail order or from a good complementary chemist.
- Buy a skin brush, Epsom salts and any oils, flower essences, foot patches or other treatments you are planning to use at home (see pages 131).
- Book appointments for complementary therapies you'd like to aid your detox methods (see page 138).

RULES OF THE 48-HOUR DETOX

- No caffeine or alcohol are allowed. Substitute herb teas, dandelion root coffee and fresh juices.
- No dairy foods are permitted. Milk and cheese increase mucus production and are difficult to digest. Lactose is a common food intolerance. You can replace milk with almond milk, rice milk, oat milk or soya milk. Sheep's and goat's products are easier to digest if you really cannot do without dairy.
- No wheat or gluten-containing grains, such as rye, which have an acid effect on the digestion. This means no bread, pasta or white rice. Choose oats, brown rice, millet and quinoa instead.
- No meat or poultry, because of the antibiotics and food additives they contain. For protein, choose plant sources, organic eggs, tofu or oily fish from organic (non-farmed) sources.

- Don't eat any processed or ready-made foods whatsoever. Everything should be fresh and cooked without salt, sugar or sweeteners. Use only fresh herbs for seasoning.
- Eat three meals and two snacks every day, making sure that you have something to eat every three hours. Most of your food will be vegetables and fruit, whole grains and plant proteins. There are sample 48-hour plans in the next chapter.
- Do make sure that you get at least 20 minutes of exercise every day, depending on what you enjoy doing, e.g. cycling, walking, jogging, swimming.
- Make sure that you drink 2 litres (3^1/$_2$ pints) of water every day and you can also have cups of herbal (non-caffeine-containing) teas whenever you feel like them.
- Dry-brush your skin before taking a shower or bath at least once a day and, if you can bear it, follow your bathing routine with a cold shower (see page 132).

When should I detox?

In Traditional Chinese Medicine, spring and summer are the best seasons for a detox. Winter is a time to rest and recuperate, eating a wholesome and warming diet. Spring is the best time to deep-cleanse the liver and gall bladder. Light, cleansing foods should be eaten in summer, and in the autumn the focus is on the intestine, lungs and skin, as you eat harvest vegetables, such as pumpkin and squash.

WHAT CAN YOU EXPECT?

Headaches and fatigue are not abnormal when you start your detox. Some people, on longer detox regimes, even feel as though they are coming down with flu, a syndrome that complementary therapists call a 'healing crisis'. What is happening is that old chemicals stored in fat tissues are being released into the bloodstream: antibiotics, pesticides, food additives, heavy metals and other waste products.

Some people break out in spots as their body sheds toxins through the skin; others get constipation, diarrhoea or bad breath with the change in digestive routine; and many may feel may giddy and nauseous. Take it easy and keep on drinking 2 litres (3$^{1}/_{2}$ pints) of water throughout the day.

Benefits

Although you won't purge a lifetime's worth of toxins during your first-ever detox, you will have made a significant difference. Next time you try a detox, the healing crisis won't be so severe and will probably not last so long. A 48-hour detox is a step towards better health, but you should find that by the end of it, your skin looks clearer and glowing, your clothes fit better, and you feel more energetic and clear-headed. Your bowels and liver should function more efficiently and you'll have given your immune system a mini-boost.

Weight loss

Detoxing is a great starting point for losing weight, and most people shed some pounds when they detox even for a short period, as they avoid the fats, sugars and processed foods and drinks that pile on the calories. If you return to your previous eating patterns, you will soon replace any weight you've lost, so if you want to go on losing weight, keep eating according to detox rules, but reintroduce organic meats and poultry, wheat and dairy gradually. Stay off processed and packaged foods and eat as many fresh foods as possible. You probably will not need to calorie-count or reduce your portions – few people overeat on such a healthy diet.

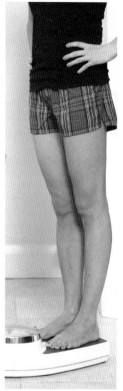

COMING OFF YOUR DETOX

Don't wolf down a four-cheese pizza and a bottle of Pinot Grigio or you will feel unwell. Keep eating the same kinds of food as on the detox but gradually introduce organic poultry, then red meat, goat's or sheep's cheese and whole grain bread.

Food intolerances

If you suspect you are intolerant to a particular food, leave five days between reintroducing each new food and watching for a reaction. If you experience bloating, headaches, skin rashes, joint pain or unusual symptoms, you may exclude the culprit from your diet for a longer period. All traces of a food will be removed from the body within two months, so reintroduce it after three months to see if it is tolerated. Sometimes intolerances pass, especially if you have been helping your system by unburdening some of the toxic load.

Kick-start the day

Some people swear by the benefits of kick-starting their system first thing in the morning with a drink of freshly squeezed lemon juice (from unwaxed organic lemons) added to hot water. Just sip it slowly and feel it cleansing your gut ready to face the day. It may precipitate the day's first bowel movement. Leave half an hour after this drink before eating your detox breakfast.

Develop good habits

Hang onto as many good habits from the detox as you can fit comfortably into your lifestyle, and try to opt for liver-supporting foods. You don't have to be rigid to be successful. For instance, if you miss coffee, you could reintroduce a single cup of organic coffee in the morning, but check for any symptoms of dependence developing, e.g. jitteriness and inability to concentrate without it. Most detox experts advise that you repeat your detox at regular intervals, say, every six months.

FASTING

Many 48-hour detox regimes generally involve fasting – cutting out food altogether and surviving on water alone, or just water plus freshly prepared fruit and vegetable juices. Some juice fasts allow you to have raw vegetables as well. You won't find many GPs or mainstream medical specialists who approve of this drastic kind of measure, and you certainly should not undertake a fast unless you are in an extremely good state of health to start with.

Don't choose fasting as your first-ever type of detox. Wait until you have tried a few of the 48-hour plans featured in this book and are no longer experiencing side effects from them. Build up gradually to a fast, as the body can go into panic mode if you suddenly make a huge change in your eating habits. If your system thinks that you are starving, it will retain all the fat (and toxins) it can, rather than releasing fat cells for elimination in the usual way.

The rules of fasting

- You can start preparing for your fast several weeks in advance, cutting out caffeine, alcohol, wheat, meat and dairy. Get used to eating mainly plant foods.
- Don't ever fast if you have any kind of chronic illness or have recently recovered from a viral or bacterial infection.
- The first time you fast, only do it for a day. Stay at home if possible because you may feel very faint and weak. You certainly shouldn't drive or operate heavy machinery.
- Drink 2–3 litres (3$^1/_2$–5 pints) of water on your fast day, and a selection of juices made from organic fruits and vegetables. Fruits are good for cleansing, while vegetables help to repair the cells.
- Don't do a water fast for longer than a day except under the supervision of a qualified health practitioner, and don't do a juice fast for longer than three days. You are not getting the nutrients you need to stay healthy and your detox will soon become counterproductive, because the liver needs protein in order to carry out its detoxification processes.
- Wean yourself gradually back onto solids after the fast has finished, starting with soups, oat porridge and easy-to-digest dishes.

HEALTHY HABITS

Even those medical specialists who disapprove of detoxing agree that it can be a valuable process if it helps to teach you more healthy habits that you retain long after the detox is over.

HEALTH BENEFITS

By retaining the healthy habits you acquire during even a brief 48-hour detox, you will experience many ongoing health benefits after you stop detoxing. For instance, you will find that you get fewer headaches and your skin will look better if you keep drinking 2 litres (3$^1/_2$ pints) of water a day. Your immune system should function more effectively if you stick with a nutritious, healthy diet that is full of antioxidant-rich

Lactose intolerance

This results from a deficiency in lactase, which is the enzyme responsible for digesting lactose in milk. It is more common in those people with certain ethnic backgrounds. It affects more than 50 per cent of people of Native American, Afro-Caribbean or Indian origins, but only three per cent of Caucasians. Young children may get temporary bouts of lactose intolerance after they've been treated with antibiotics or had a dose of gastroenteritis.

Food combining

Some nutritionists believe that it is easier for our digestive systems to break down foods if we don't eat a protein and a carbohydrate at the same meal. It is worth trying if you suffer from digestive problems. Eat protein and salad or vegetables for one meal a day, then eat grains, pasta or cereals with vegetables for another, and only eat fruit on its own at least 30 minutes after a meal.

fruits and vegetables, and you will have a better chance of avoiding heart disease and several types of cancer.

You should try to keep your fibre intake up at around 35g a day for healthy bowel function and to protect you against the increasingly common colon cancer. Keep skin brushing to hold the cellulite at bay and you will improve your circulation all round. Also, by cutting out the junk foods in your diet, you will lose some weight and have a much better chance of keeping your weight within a healthy band for your height and age.

Mini-detoxes

Mini-detoxes, where you follow the 48-hour plans in this book or just give up alcohol or caffeine for a week without necessarily following the other rules, can give your health a valuable boost. They teach you good long-term habits for the future, and you can repeat your mini-detoxes several times a year.

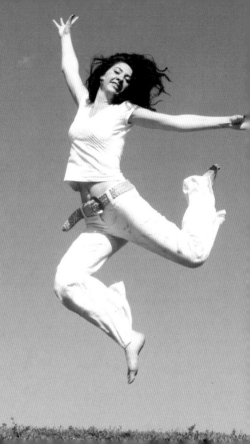

PART 3

Detox guidelines

Detoxing isn't just about avoiding the foods and drinks that tax the liver and burden the digestive system; it's also about opting for fresh, natural foods that positively boost your metabolism and provide loads of health-promoting nutrients that strengthen your natural detoxification processes. The main aim of the diet is not weight loss, so do not start counting calories or jumping on the scales every day. The benefits will be measured in how well you look and feel at the end of your detox programme.

CLEAN UP YOUR DIET

You should never go hungry when you are detoxing. Eat as much as you like. Have between-meal snacks. The only rule is that you stick to detox foods and drinks. If you have stocked your store cupboards and fridge in advance, it should not be too hard.

GO ORGANIC

What is the point of going to a lot of trouble to cleanse the toxins from your system if you are simultaneously reintroducing new ones with every morsel you eat? By choosing organically grown foods, you can avoid the most harmful pesticides. The ones that are used on organic crops are strictly regulated, and natural farming methods are used to control pests, including crop rotation and the planting of anti-pest plants alongside crops. Look for the organic certification logo on the products you buy in supermarkets and food stores.

Money tight?

If you cannot afford to buy all organic, at the very least avoid the fruits and vegetables with the biggest toxin load when they are grown conventionally: strawberries, apples, cherries, apricots, blackberries, pears, raspberries, peaches, imported grapes, spinach, peppers, celery and potatoes.

Harmful chemicals

Some fruit and vegetable crops are treated with more harmful chemicals than others:

● Non-organic strawberries are covered in captan, a fungicide that has been linked to cancer, and damage to the immune, nervous and reproductive systems.

● Non-organic apples contain diphenylamine, which some experts believe causes brain and nervous system damage, and thiabendazole, which may damage the reproductive system.

● Non-organic celery contains permethrin, chlorothalonil and acephate, which have all been linked to cancer.

● Non-organic spinach may have up to 40 harmful pesticides on its leaves.

Preparing fruit and vegetables

No amount of washing or peeling will shift these chemicals as the soil they were grown and nurtured in is replete with toxins. Wash and peel them, but do not kid yourself that you are solving the problem.

Organic certification

Be careful when buying so-called 'organic' and 'pure' products. Always check that they carry the symbol of the Soil Association or another certifying body, to be sure their organic purity has been verified and that the product has been produced and processed according to strict and rigorous environmental and animal welfare standards.

IS ORGANIC MORE NUTRITIOUS?

Researchers at John Hopkins University looked at the results of 41 studies over a 50-year period and they concluded that, on average, organic food contained 30 per cent more vitamin C, over 20 per cent more iron, 30 per cent more magnesium and 14 per cent more phosphorus than conventionally grown food, as well as 15 per cent fewer harmful nitrates.

Meat and poultry

Although you will not eat meat on your detox, it is worth knowing that organically reared animals cannot be fed the growth enhancers and parasiticides that non-organic animals receive. Antibiotics are not given preventively and, if the animal becomes ill and requires antibiotic treatment, it is removed from the organic herd. Their feed must be 100 per cent organic, with no genetically modified ingredients and no animal by-products. Finally, when the meat is sold, it should contain no artificial ingredients, food colourings or chemical preservatives.

Without going into gruesome details, pork is probably the most toxic of non-organic meats because pigs don't sweat out toxins in the same way as some other animals. Non-organic chicken can be bad for your health with more than 60 per cent of factory-farmed birds infected with campylobacter from their own faeces, and more than 30 per cent infected with salmonella.

HELP YOUR LIVER TO DETOX

Foods from the brassica family (cabbage, cauliflower, kale, pak choi, broccoli and Brussels sprouts) contain phytonutrients which are essential to the liver's detoxification processes and help the liver convert fat-soluble toxins into water-soluble substances which can be passed from the body in urine.

LIVER HEALERS

Sulphur-rich foods, such as garlic, onions, eggs and red peppers, help the liver to eliminate toxins in a process called sulphation. In Asian restaurants, you may be served a long, white radish called a Daikon after eating particularly fatty foods, because its high sulphur content helps the body to metabolize and digest fats. Certain other foods, some of which are listed in the following pages, are powerful liver healers because

Beating the booze

If you know you drink too much, it's best to stay away from other drinkers when you give up alcohol to help you resist temptation. Follow the advice on healing your liver, drink dandelion root tea and coffee, and take some milk thistle (see page 123) and a good multivitamin supplement. Contact Alcoholics Anonymous if you have trouble giving up.

they contain key ingredients, and these should all be part of your detox programme. There are also a number of herbal supplements that boost liver function and will aid an effective detox (see page 122).

Artichoke hearts

These aid the secretion of bile, containing antioxidants, which are known as flavonoids, protecting the liver cells. Artichokes are useful for people with alcohol-related liver problems, and they are also a fantastic detox aid.

Asparagus

This delicious seasonal vegetable is a good source of vitamin A and potassium, which the liver needs to detox. Asparagus is also rich in folate, vitamin E and fibre, so try to include it in your diet.

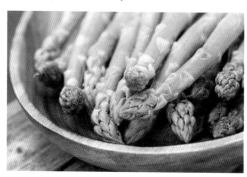

Beetroot

This contains betaine, which protects the liver from alcohol. Beetroot also thins the bile and helps it to flow along the bile ducts more easily.

Dandelion roots

Dandelion roots contain inulin, which nourishes beneficial gut bacteria, stimulates liver function, and helps to lower blood sugar. You can buy dandelion tea and coffee in most health food shops.

B vitamins

Contained in whole grains and pulses, such as oats, millet, chickpeas and brown rice, the B vitamins are essential in a liver detox. Vitamin B1 helps us to deal with the effects of alcohol, smoking and heavy metals. Vitamin B2 is used to produce glutathione. Vitamin B3 is needed for the breakdown of several toxins, whereas vitamin B4 detoxifies the acetaldehyde byproduct of alcohol breakdown.

Seeds

Pumpkin, sunflower, sesame, flax and alfalfa seeds are a concentrated source of vitamins, minerals and essential fatty acids. You can toast pumpkin and sunflower seeds in the oven to bring out the flavour, or soak the seeds in water before eating to make them easier to digest. Sprinkle them on soups, salads, stir-fries or casseroles, or on your breakfast cereal.

Magnesium

This essential mineral is found in dark green, leafy foods and is one of the key nutrients your liver needs to manufacture enzymes for toxin breakdown. Choose bitter green leaves, such as watercress, rocket, chard, dandelion greens or mustard greens, to help your digestive enzymes and to provide the chlorophyll which purifies the blood.

Oranges, lemons and limes

All these citrus fruits stimulate the production of glutathione and help the process by which the body eliminates sulpha drugs. So start finding some new ways to use them; here are some ideas to help you. Why not add some lemon juice to a cup of hot water to start the day? Or you could try mixing it with olive oil instead of vinegar as a salad dressing; or squeezing some fresh orange and lime juice over a variety of crisp, wok-fried vegetables.

Seaweed

Vegetables that come from the sea contain more minerals than any other single food source, with 10 times as much calcium as milk, and eight times as much iron as you'll find in beef. Choose arame, nori, wakame, kelp, kombu, dulse and hijiki. Follow the cooking instructions on the pack or just throw some strips into the pot when you're cooking beans, rice or casseroles.

Turmeric

The key spice found in curries, giving them their distinctive yellow colour as well as flavour, turmeric slows down the first stage of detoxification in the liver but speeds up the second, so that you are less prone to damage from the intermediate toxic chemicals and their associated free radicals.

LIVE YOGHURT

Live yoghurt is a superfood that contains probiotics: the beneficial bacteria that displace harmful toxins in your intestine. However, you must be sure that you get the right kind, which has a high lactobacilli content. Always check the label when you are buying pots of yoghurt; it should say that it is 'made with live and active cultures'. If it has been frozen, or has had artificial colours and fruit flavours added, then you are on the wrong track.

Probiotic bacteria

These are fragile, and those that are found in so-called 'bio' yoghurt which has been standing around on a supermarket shelf or in your fridge for a week or more will contain fewer live bacteria than freshly made cultures. If you are in doubt, then you can buy probiotic supplements in most health food shops – select one that supplies at least 1–2 billion colony-forming units (CFU) of acidophilus per dose.

WHAT KIND OF WATER?

Our blood is 83 per cent water, and it needs its supply of water to keep being replenished if it is to get rid of all the toxins and waste products that your cells are shedding during a detox programme. But what kind of water should you drink?

IS TAP WATER GOOD FOR YOU?

Concerns about tap water include the risk of lead poisoning if your house was built before the 1970s and has lead piping. Even if it has been replumbed, the stop valve could be made of lead. Even low levels of lead in the system have been linked by some studies to miscarriages in pregnant women, brain damage in children and poisoning in adults. If you think that there might be lead in your water, then contact the Drinking Water Inspectorate (see page 184).

According to some studies, adding fluoride to water suppresses thyroid function and causes the organs to

Buying water filters

You can look in your local directory for water treatment equipment suppliers, or ask your plumber to install a filter on your cold tap. For more water filter information and sales advice, see opposite.

stockpile aluminium, but several areas in the UK still add it to the water supply to help protect against tooth decay. To find out what's in your local supply, you can ask for a water quality report from your local supplier.

FILTRATION SYSTEMS

You can now purchase several different kinds of water filtration systems to remove the contaminants from your tap water. Here are the most popular ones.

Jug filters

These remove lime scale, chlorine and other impurities, but not hormones, fluoride or nitrates. The greatest improvement is taste, not quality. The filters should be changed monthly to be effective.

Plumbed-in sink filters

Manufacturers of plumbed-in sink filters claim that they remove heavy metals, chlorine and 80 per cent of bacteria and pesticides. Once you have got past the installation cost, these filters are cheaper to run and more efficient than jug filters.

Reverse osmosis filters

The King of Filters is the reverse osmosis filter, filtering out between 95 and 98 per cent of minerals, chemicals, metals and bacteria, and thereby leaving you with a product that is purer than many bottled waters.

How pure is your water?

It is quite frightening to think about how many toxins are present in our ordinary tap water. Below is an example of all the contaminating substances that just one reverse osmosis filter can remove in the purification process. You can see why it is a good investment for your health and an important detox aid.

Bacteria 95%+	Chlorine 95%+
Endrin 95%+	Chromate 85–90%
Glucose 95%+	Copper 94–97%
Lindane 95%+	Cyanide 85–90%
Methoxychlor 95%+	Hardness 93–96%
Phenol 95%+	Iron 94–97%
Protein 95%+	Lead 95%+
Pyrogens 95%+	Magnesium 93–96%
Sucrose 95%+	Mercury 94–97%
THM's 95%+	Nickel 94–97%
Toxaphene 95%+	Nitrate 50–90%
Urea 95%+	Phosphate 97%
Virus 95%+	Potassium 88–82%
Aluminium 97%	Silicate 88–93%
Ammonium 85–90%	Silver 88–92%
Bicarbonate 91–95%	Sodium 88–92%
Bromide 88–92%	Strontium 93–96%
Cadmium 93–96%	Sulphate 93–96%
Calcium 93–96%	Zinc 94–97%
Chloride 88–92%	Fluoride 95%

How many times do you go?

When you increase your water intake to the recommended 2 litres (3½ pints) a day, or 8 x 125ml (4fl oz) glasses, you'll find yourself trotting backwards and forwards to the loo more frequently than usual, but within a week your system will grow accustomed to the extra liquid intake.

Bottled mineral water

This is convenient when you're out and about during the day. Buy it in bulk in supermarkets or purchase one from a newsagent or vending machine. Mineral water can get contaminated, so check the product is within its sell-by date to avoid the risk of antimony poisoning from polyethylene terephthalate (PET) bottles. If you buy larger glass bottles, you can recycle them..

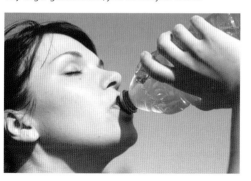

DETOX SHOPPING LIST

If there are chocolate biscuits stored at the back of the cupboard or some chilled Chardonnay in the fridge, then the chances are that you'll succumb during a weak moment and, no matter how good your initial intentions, you will break your detox.

So before you start your detox, make sure you clear out any 'banned' foods. Give them away to your friends or family, and replace them with delicious detox foods to give you the best chance of success.

FOODS TO AVOID

It is so easy when you are pushing your trolley up and down the aisles of the supermarket to be tempted by all sorts of attractively packaged unhealthy and junk foods and to pop them in. However, you must learn to harden your resolve and opt for the healthy foods listed in the shopping list opposite while avoiding the foods featured below.

Don't eat the following:

• Wheat products: including bread, wheat-based breakfast cereals, pasta, flour, noodles (except rice noodles), couscous, cakes, biscuits and pizza.

• Processed foods: including ready meals, ready-made

sauces, condiments, stock cubes (unless organic), potato crisps, desserts, spreads, and anything that contains artificial additives. Always check the labels if you are unsure.

• Dairy products: including milk, cow's cheese, cream, butter and normal, non-live yoghurts.
• All meat, poultry, game and non-organic fish.
• Caffeine: including black or green tea, coffee, colas and other fizzy drinks, chocolate and painkillers.
• Sugars: including sweets, squashes, cordials and any fruit juices except freshly squeezed.
• Alcohol.

Your detox shopping list

Fruits

Apples	Kiwi	Peaches
Apricots	Lemons	Pears
Avocado	Limes	Pineapple
Blackberries	Lychees	Plums
Blackcurrants	Mango	Pomegranate
Blueberries	Melon	Raspberries
Cherries	Nectarines	Strawberries
Greengages	Oranges	
	Papaya	

Vegetables

Artichokes	Aubergine	Cabbage
(canned and	Beetroot	Carrots
fresh)	Broccoli	Cauliflower
Asparagus	Butternut	Celery
	squash	Courgettes

Continued on page 72

Your detox shopping list continued…

Cucumber
Green beans
Leeks
Mange-tout
Onions
Peas
Peppers
Pumpkins

Rocket
Salad greens
Spinach
Spring greens
Squash
Sweet potatoes
Sweetcorn
Swiss chard

Tomatoes (canned
    and fresh)
Watercress
All kind of fresh
    herbs: basil, mint,
    parsley,
    coriander, etc.

Grains	corn, quinoa, rice	noodles
Amaranth	or millet	Whole oat flakes
Brown rice	Quinoa	Wheatgrass, barley
Buckwheat	Rice noodles	grass, alfalfa
Millet	Rye flakes	grass
Pasta made from	Soba (buckwheat)	Wild rice

Pulses (dried or canned)	Broad beans	Haricot beans
	Butter beans	Lentils, red or
Adzuki beans	Cannelini beans	green
Black-eye beans	Chickpeas	Red kidney beans
Black beans	Flageolet beans	Sprouted beans

Nuts and seeds	Coconuts	Pine nuts
Almonds	Dried fruit	Pumpkin seeds
Brazil nuts	(unsulphured)	Sesame seeds
Cashews	Flax seeds	Sunflower seeds
Chestnuts	Hazelnuts	Walnuts

Breads and crispbreads	Wheat-free, yeast-free bread	Rice cakes
	Oatcakes	Rye crackers

Spreads and dips	Hummus	fats)
Guacamole	Nut butters (no	Tahini
Honey	hydrogenated	

Protein	Organic oily fish	Seaweed
Organic free-range	(salmon,	(wakame, nori,
eggs	mackerel,	arami, kelp,
Goat's or sheep's	herring,	kombu, dulse,
cheese,	sardines)	hijiki)
including feta	Live natural	
cheese and	yoghurt	
mozzarella	Tofu and tempeh	

Oils and fats	Flaxseed oil	Pumpkin seed oil
Extra-virgin	Sesame seed oil	
olive oil	Walnut oil	

Spices and	Ginger	sauces rather
flavourings	Hot pepper sauce	than soy, which
Balsamic vinegar	Japanese rice	can contain
Chillies	vinegar	caramel and
Cider vinegar	Lemongrass	wheat
Cumin	Paprika	Turmeric
Garlic	Shoyu or tamari	

Drinks	Herbal teas of your	almond, rice,
Water filters or	choice	sesame, soya)
bottles of still,	Non-dairy,	
low-sodium	calcium- fortified	
mineral water	milk (e.g.	

JUICING

It is well worth buying a juicer, whether you are on a detox or not, just for the megadoses of vitamins and minerals that fresh juice can deliver in one hit. You will not get the same benefits from shop-bought 'freshly squeezed' juices; orange juice, for example, starts to lose its vitamin content seven minutes after being squeezed.

HAVE FUN EXPERIMENTING

You don't get all the fibre of the fruit and vegetables when you juice them, but the vitamin content is more than you would get otherwise because who would eat eight oranges in one sitting? However, a large glass of juice might contain the juice of eight oranges.

Buy a juicer with a removeable filter so you don't have to clean the whole mechanism every time you use it. Buy organic fruit and vegetables, and clean, peel, deseed and chop them before putting them in the juicer. Experiment with your favourite ingredients to come up with your own recipes, or try the following:

Veg-based combinations

- 3 carrots, 2 fennel stalks and $1/2$ lemon
- 3 carrots, 2 celery stalks, 2cm (1in) fresh root ginger and $1/2$ apple

- 3–4 carrots, 1–2 celery stalks and a small wedge of cabbage
- 1 green pepper, 1 red pepper, 3 celery stalks, $1/2$ cucumber and 5 lettuce leaves
- 5 handfuls spinach, 1 cucumber and 2 carrots
- 1 beetroot, 2 carrots, a small handful of spinach, 2 tomatoes and a squeeze of fresh lime juice
- 5 carrots, 1 apple and $1/2$ beetroot
- $1/2$ head of broccoli, a handful each of watercress and parsley, 1 stick of celery and $1/2$ fresh pineapple
- 4–5 carrots, $1/2$ lemon, 1 apple, small wedge of red cabbage and a small piece of fresh root ginger
- 3 celery stalks, a handful of spinach, 2 asparagus stalks and 1 large tomato
- A large leaf each of kale and collard, a handful of parsley, 1 celery stalk, 1 carrot, $1/2$ red pepper, 1 tomato and 1 large broccoli floret

Fruit-based combinations

- 2 apples, 2 pears and 2cm (1in) fresh root ginger
- A handful of blueberries, handful of raspberries, 1 apple and 2 nectarines
- 1 orange, 1 mango and 1 kiwi fruit
- 12 strawberries and 4–5 carrots
- A large slice of watermelon, a cup of ripe strawberries and the juice and zest of 1 lime
- 2 oranges, 4 carrots and 2cm (1in) fresh root ginger
- A large bunch of seedless grapes, 1 apple and some fresh mint leaves

SMOOTHIES

To turn your fruit-based juice into a smoothie is not difficult. All you need do is just add some live natural yoghurt and then whizz together in a food processor or blender until smooth. Alternatively, for a healthy fruit-based milkshake, you can add a non-dairy soya, rice or almond milk – although note that none of these would be allowed on a juice-based fast.

Detox tip: You should always drink your freshly squeezed juices, smoothies and shakes immediately in order to gain the maximum nutritional value.

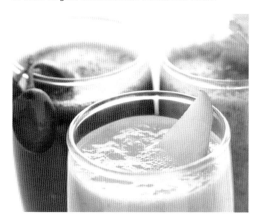

TIME FOR TEA

You can drink any herbal teas you fancy on a detox, but the ones featured here have special benefits to help cleanse the system. Many of the tea manufacturers now make their own 'Detox' or 'Cleansing' brands, which will often contain a mixture of useful ingredients, but you should always buy organic teas if you can.

SUITABLE TEAS

Decaff coffee and tea are not recommended on a detox diet because of the methods that are used to extract the caffeine. The methylene chloride that is used in some decaffeinating processes is related to the toxic perchlorethylene used in dry cleaning. An organic solvent called ethyl acetate is also sometimes used, and the product might be labelled 'naturally decaffeinated' because this chemical occurs in some fruits and in the coffee itself, but studies have shown that it is still highly

Dandelion root coffee

Buy dandelion roots from a health food shop and allow them to dry. Place the dried roots on a baking tray in an oven preheated to 200°C, Gas Mark 6 and roast them until they are a deep brown colour. Store in a glass jar and when you are ready to use, grind them into a fine powder using a coffee mill. Add a teaspoon to a cup of boiling water, stir and then drink.

toxic. Try a few of the following teas to see which one you prefer – they all taste different and have specific properties, and it is a matter of personal taste which you choose to drink.

Which tea?

- Nettle tea is a diuretic, meaning it helps your body to excrete water, so it will flush out your toxins more quickly.
- Milk thistle tea contains silymarin which makes the liver less susceptible to toxin damage and increases its production of glutathione.
- Red sorrel tea is a terrific liver and gall bladder cleanser, and a recent study has indicated that it decreases the blood triglyceride levels (high levels are associated with heart disease and diabetes).
- Dandelion leaf tea has a diuretic action, while dandelion root coffee is an effective detox aid, stimulating the flow of bile so that more toxins are

Leaf tea

The herbal teabags you buy are absolutely fine, but once you have tried making your own brew from fresh leaves there will be no going back. A big handful of mint leaves, steeped in boiling water for 5 minutes, makes the most delicious mint tea. Some health food shops sell herbal preparations that you can use to make your own teas, and will invariably provide more taste than the powdered preparations that are used in teabags.

eliminated through the bowels.

- Rooibosch (or Red Bush) tea helps you to shed toxins through sweat, can relieve bloating and also aid the digestive process. It is claimed to reduce the effects of ageing, keep the skin, teeth and bones healthy, and it can aid sleep.
- Chamomile tea is calming, soporific and can help to relieve mild headaches.
- Lemon balm helps with depression and anxiety.
- Spearmint and peppermint tea both aid digestion.
- Fennel tea stimulates the liver.

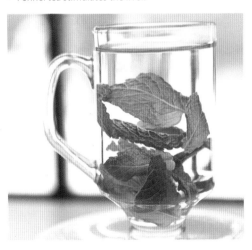

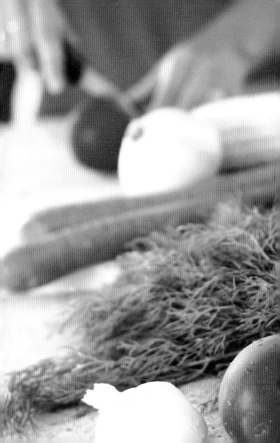

PART 4

48-hour detox plans

Here are eight 48-hour detox plans to suit every taste. You can choose what you want for breakfast, lunch, dinner and snacks from the options given. There are easy-to-follow recipes within each plan. You should try to keep the ingredients varied and make sure you eat a range of different-coloured fruits and vegetables every day. These healthy eating plans will help your clothes to fit better and make you feel generally more energetic and more comfortable about yourself.

MENU PLANS

Choose what you want each day for breakfast, lunch, dinner and snacks, so long as you keep the ingredients varied and try to eat a range of different-coloured fruits and vegetables every day.

Breakfast choices

On every plan featured in the following pages, you can choose one of the following breakfasts:

- Oat porridge made with whole oats (not instant) and served with non-dairy milk, honey and nuts
- Millet or quinoa porridge with a dried fruit topping, served with non-dairy milk
- Compôte of mixed dried fruits soaked in orange juice and served with live yoghurt
- Non-wheat bread toasted and served with nut butter or honey
- Poached organic eggs and steamed spinach on non-wheat toast
- Fruit salad of mango, papaya and melon topped with sesame seeds
- Start-the-day cereal (see opposite)

Start-the-day cereal (serves 1)

Ingredients

4–5 dsp whole oat flakes
1–2 dsp sunflower seeds
1–2 dsp pumpkin seeds
4–5 Brazil nuts or 6–8 other
    unsalted nuts
½ dessertspoon organic
    dried fruit (this may not
    be necessary if your fresh

fruit is sweet enough)
non-dairy soya, almond
    or rice milk
fresh fruit in season, e.g.
    strawberries, raspberries,
    chopped mango, peach,
    pear, apple, gooseberries,
    blueberries

Just mix all the ingredients together. This cereal will provide you with a good dose of fibre, B vitamins, iron, magnesium, zinc, omega-3 and omega-6 fatty acids from the seeds, protein and minerals from the nuts, and vitamin C from the fruit. Adjust the quantities according to appetite and preference.

The oat flakes are easiest to digest if you soak them in the milk for a couple of hours (or leave them overnight in the fridge). Toasting in a hot oven or dry-frying brings out the flavour of the sunflower and pumpkin seeds. But if you're in a hurry, as most of us are in the morning, just mix the ingredients in a bowl and eat.

Plan 1

Breakfast choices
See page 82

Lunch choices
- Spinach and garlic soup, with non-wheat bread
- Salad leaves with tomatoes, cucumber, peppers, a slice of goat's cheese and walnuts sprinkled on top with a little vinaigrette dressing

Dinner choices
- A selection of roasted vegetables, e.g. beetroot, aubergine, courgette, tomatoes and red onion, with pumpkin seeds and crumbled feta cheese on top
- Baked organic salmon (preferably wild) with your vegetable accompaniment of choice
- Oriental stir-fried broccoli (see page 86)

Dessert choices
- Any kind of fresh fruit salad
- Pomegranate ice (see page 87)

Snacks
- Any fresh fruit – melon, grapes, apple, pear, satsuma
- A fresh juice, smoothie or non-dairy milk shake

Spinach and garlic soup (Serves 2)

Ingredients

1 small onion, chopped
1 tsp olive oil
2 garlic cloves, chopped
handful of chopped parsley
225g (8oz) fresh spinach,
    chopped

400ml (14fl oz) vegetable
    stock *or* water
juice of 1/2 lemon
salt and black pepper
grated nutmeg (optional)
sprigs of parsley, to garnish

1 Soften the onion in the olive oil gently, without burning, for 5 minutes. Add the garlic and cook slowly until both are soft. Add the parsley and the spinach; you may need to add the latter in batches, waiting as it cooks down before adding more.

2 Add the water or vegetable stock and cook gently for 10 minutes maximum. The spinach should still be green; if it begins to change colour before the time is up, remove the pan from the heat immediately.

3 Stir in the lemon juice and allow the soup to cool a little. Blend, adjusting the consistency if wished by adding a little more liquid. Check the seasoning, reheat gently and add a little grated nutmeg (optional). Serve garnished with parsley.

Oriental stir-fried broccoli (serves 1)

Ingredients

10g (⅓ oz) sesame seeds

10g (⅓ oz) cashew nuts

1 tsp sesame oil

4 radishes, sliced diagonally

4 large spring onions, sliced diagonally

½ red pepper, seeded and chopped

½ yellow pepper, seeded and chopped

2.5cm (1in) root ginger, peeled and chopped

½ red chilli, seeded and finely chopped

1 garlic clove, chopped

200g (7oz) purple sprouting broccoli florets

dash of shoyu or light soy sauce

salt and black pepper

1 Dry-roast the sesame seeds and cashew nuts in a dry frying pan. When they smell really toasted and colour up, remove the pan from the heat and set aside.

2 Heat the sesame oil in a wok, and add the radishes, spring onions and peppers. Stir-fry for 2 minutes, then add the ginger, chilli and garlic. When the peppers begin to soften, add the broccoli and stir-fry for a few more minutes. Add a dash of shoyu or light soy sauce and cook until the broccoli begins to soften – it should retain some crunch. Stir in the cashews and sesame seeds. Check the seasoning, and serve immediately.

Pomegranate ice (serves 1)

Ingredients

½ large pomegranate,
  or 1 whole smaller one
6 ice cubes

1 tbsp water
1 tsp orange flower water

1 Squeeze the pomegranate upside-down over a bowl to catch the juice and loosen the seeds. Whack the skin with the back of a wooden spoon, so the seeds fall into the bowl. Squeeze the skin again to extract as much juice as possible, and discard. Remove any small pieces of pith from the bowl containing the seeds and juice.

2 Put the ice cubes in a blender with the water and crush, using the pulse setting – alternatively, place in a self-seal plastic bag, close it and hit with a rolling pin. Make a mound of crushed ice in a serving dish (this looks wonderful in a glass bowl) and scatter the pomegranate seeds and juice over the top; the ice will turn a delicate pale garnet colour in parts. Drizzle the orange flower water over everything and serve.

Tip: If you can't get hold of orange flower water, you can use fresh orange juice instead.

Plan 2

Breakfast choices
See page 82

Lunch choices
• Warm asparagus salad
• Non-wheat pasta with steamed vegetables and a simple tomato sauce made by cooking garlic, chopped onion, herbs and tomatoes in olive oil

Dinner choices
• Grilled or baked mackerel, served with heaps of seasonal vegetables and a squeeze of lemon juice
• Pasta with artichokes (see page 90)

Dessert choices
• Any kind of fresh fruit salad
• Orange and date salad (see page 91)

Snacks
• Any fresh fruit – melon, grapes, apple, pear, satsuma
• A fresh juice, smoothie or non-dairy milk shake
• Rice cakes (unsalted, plain or sesame seed), oatcakes or non-wheat bread with hummus, tahini, guacamole, goat's cheese, nut butter or honey

Warm asparagus salad (serves 1)

Ingredients

6–10 hazelnuts, chopped
250g (8oz) bunch of
   asparagus, timmed
1/2 large courgette
handful of salad leaves
salt and black pepper

For the dressing:

1/2 tsp Dijon mustard
1/2 tsp clear honey
juice of 1/2 small lemon
1 tsp olive oil

1 Dry-roast the nuts in a non-stick pan; when they start to smell toasted, remove the pan from the heat.

2 Cook the asparagus in a pan of boiling water for 3 minutes. Make long strips of courgette with a potato peeler. Add to the asparagus and cook for 1 minute.

3 Whisk the dressing ingredients together until smooth. Arrange the salad leaves on a plate.

4 Drain and allow to cool briefly until the asparagus can be handled, and then arrange both the asparagus pieces and the courgette strips on top of the salad leaves. Whisk the dressing once more and drizzle it over everything, season with salt and black pepper and scatter the hazelnuts on top. Serve immediately.

Pasta with artichokes (serves 1)

Ingredients

75g (3oz) wheat-free pasta,
   (dry weight)
1 tsp olive oil
1 garlic clove, chopped
5 pieces of artichoke from

a jar of artichokes in olive
   oil, drained and chopped
6 olives, chopped
chopped flat-leaved parsley
salt and black pepper

1 Bring a pan of water to a rolling boil, then add the pasta. Cook for about 6–8 minutes, or according to the instructions on the packet.

2 When the pasta is nearly done, warm the olive oil in a frying pan and add the garlic. When it begins to colour, stir in the chopped artichokes and olives and warm them through.

3 Drain the pasta, then return it to the pan, and add the artichokes, olives and garlic from the frying pan. Season with salt and black pepper, and stir in the chopped parsley. Serve immediately.

Tip: Artichokes contain flavonoids that protect liver cells and aid the secretion of bile which helps us to digest fats. All in all, they are a class A detox food.

Orange and date salad (serves 1)

Ingredients
1 large juicy orange   4 dates

1 Peel the orange with a knife over a bowl, removing all the pith but catching as much juice as you can. Slice the orange flesh neatly into rounds. Slice the dates crosswise, quite finely.

2 Put a few orange slices in a dish and scatter some dates over them, then add another layer of oranges. Sprinkle the remaining dates over the top, pushing them down among the oranges.

3 Pour over the orange juice. Cover and set aside for at least 2 hours; in hot weather, store in the fridge, but bring back to room temperature before serving.

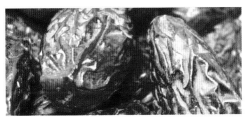

Plan 3

Breakfast choices
See page 82

Lunch choices
- Detox 'coleslaw' with seeds
- A Mediterranean vegetable two-egg omelette, with sautéed onion, courgette and peppers

Dinner choices
- Grilled sardines, served with heaps of seasonal vegetables and a squeeze of lemon juice
- Spicy bean casserole, served with brown rice and a mixed salad (see page 94)

Dessert choices
Choose one of the following:
- Any kind of fresh fruit salad
- Blueberry salad (see page 95)

Snacks
- Any fresh fruit – melon, grapes, apple, pear, satsuma
- A fresh juice, smoothie or non-dairy milk shake
- Half an avocado sprinkled with olive oil and balsamic vinegar dressing

Detox 'coleslaw' with seeds (serves 2)

Ingredients

75g (3oz) white cabbage, finely shredded

2 carrots, grated

1/2 yellow pepper, seeded and finely chopped

1 red onion, finely chopped

6 black olives, chopped

1 tsp pumpkin seeds

1 tsp sunflower seeds

For the dressing:

1 tbsp apple juice

1 tsp olive oil

1/2 tsp Dijon mustard

1 tsp lemon juice

salt and black pepper

1 Put the cabbage, carrots, yellow pepper, onions and olives in a large bowl.

2 Put all the dressing ingredients in a jar, make sure the lid is screwed on tightly, and shake well. Taste and adjust the seasoning, then pour over the vegetables and stir well.

3 Dry-roast the pumpkin and sunflower seeds in a dry frying pan, stirring them so they don't catch too much. Remove the pan from the heat as soon as they begin to colour.

4 Put the coleslaw on a serving plate and scatter the seeds on top. Serve immediately.

Spicy bean casserole (serves 2)

Ingredients

75g (3oz) dried cannellini
  beans
1 tsp olive oil
2 red onions, chopped
1 garlic clove, chopped
½ tsp ground cumin
½ tsp ground coriander
1 red chilli, chopped

water or vegetable stock
2 large tomatoes, chopped
1 red pepper, seeded and
  chopped
½ tsp paprika
2 tsp tomato purée
2 tsp organic honey
salt and black pepper

1 Soak the cannellini beans overnight. Drain and rinse, then boil in fresh water for 10 minutes. Drain again.

2 Heat the oil and cook the onions gently. Add the garlic, cumin, coriander and chilli. Cook briefly, stirring, then add the beans and cover with water or stock to a depth of 5cm (2in). Simmer for 30 minutes.

3 Add the tomatoes, red pepper, paprika, tomato purée and honey. Simmer gently for 30 minutes until well reduced; add a little more liquid if it is vanishing too quickly. Alternatively, turn the heat up to reduce it if you have too much; either way, you should end up with a thick sauce. Check the seasoning and serve with brown rice and salad.

Blueberry salad (serves 1)

Ingredients
75g (3oz) blueberries
1 kiwi fruit

10 black seedless grapes
2 slices of lime

1 Pick over the blueberries and remove any bits of stalk, then wash and drain well. Peel and thinly slice the kiwi fruit and put it in a serving bowl with the blueberries.

2 Wash the grapes, slice into rounds and scatter over the kiwi and blueberries. Squeeze one slice of lime into the bowl, then cover and chill in the refrigerator for 30 minutes. Serve, garnished with the other piece of lime.

Tip: this is an antioxidant cocktail *par excellence,* the green and purplish-black colours look very attractive.

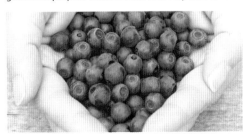

Plan 4

Breakfast choices
See page 82

Lunch choices
• Chickpea and tomato soup, served with non-wheat bread (see opposite)
• Lentil and roast pepper salad (see page 98)

Dinner choices
• Poached organic salmon served with heaps of seasonal vegetables and a squeeze of lemon juice
• Marinated vegetable kebabs, served with brown rice and green salad (see page 99)
• Grilled vegetable stack (sliced aubergine, tomato and courgettes) with grilled tofu and salad

Dessert choices
• Any kind of fresh fruit salad
• Any fresh fruit topped with home-made crumble mixture of oats and crushed nuts baked in oven

Snacks
• Any fresh fruit – melon, grapes, apple, pear, satsuma
• A fresh juice, smoothie or non-dairy milk shake
• Cherry tomatoes with chunks of goat's cheese

Chickpea and tomato soup (serves 2)

Ingredients

60g (2oz) dried chickpeas
1 tsp olive oil
1 onion, chopped
2 garlic cloves, finely
   chopped
2 courgettes (1 green and
   1 yellow, if possible),
   sliced and quartered

1 x 200g (7oz) can organic
   chopped tomatoes
water or vegetable stock
½ tsp dried Italian herb
   mix
fresh herbs, e.g. basil,
   marjoram, oregano,
   to garnish

1 Soak the chickpeas overnight. Rinse and drain them, put into fresh water and boil for 10 minutes, removing any froth that forms. Drain and rinse.

2 Warm the olive oil in a large saucepan with a lid. Add the onion and cook until translucent, then add the garlic and cook for 2 minutes, stirring. Add the courgettes and stir for 1–2 minutes.

3 Stir in the chickpeas, tomatoes and enough liquid to cover everything. Add the dried herbs and then cook gently until the chickpeas are tender, about 25 minutes, depending on how fresh they are. Serve the soup in bowls, garnished with a few fresh herb leaves.

Lentil and roast pepper salad (serves 1)

Ingredients

1 large red pepper, halved
   and seeded
a little olive oil
60g (2oz) green lentils,
   e.g. Le Puy, rinsed well
½ red onion, chopped
salad leaves

parsley, to garnish

For the dressing:

2 tsp balsamic vinegar
   (or lemon juice)
1 tsp olive oil
¼ tsp Dijon mustard

1 Rub the outside of each pepper half with olive oil and roast, cut side down, in the oven at 200°C/Gas Mark 6 for 15–20 minutes until the skins begin to blister. Cool.

2 Cook the lentils in boiling water for about 20 minutes, until soft. Drain and place in a large bowl.

3 Whisk the dressing ingredients together. Pour most of the dressing over the lentils while they are warm, add the onion and stir thoroughly.

4 Skin the peppers and cut the flesh into strips. Add to the lentils, mixing them in gently. Arrange the salad leaves on a plate, drizzle the remaining dressing over them and put the lentils and peppers in the middle. Garnish with parsley and serve immediately.

Marinated vegetable kebabs (serves 1)

Ingredients

1 tbsp shoyu or soy sauce
1 tsp sesame oil
1 tsp clear honey
1 garlic clove, crushed
1 small courgette, sliced

1 small red onion, cut into pieces
1 yellow or red pepper, cut into chunks
6–9 button mushrooms

1 Put the shoyu, sesame oil, honey and garlic in a jug and stir well. Toss all the vegetables in the marinade. Leave to marinate for 1 hour or so.

2 Preheat the grill or a barbecue. Thread the vegetables on to 3 skewers, transferring any remaining marinade into a small pan (if you don't have much left, don't worry – use some plain shoyu for dipping instead).

3 Place the kebabs under the grill or on the barbecue and cook, being careful to turn them regularly. Warm the remaining marinade over a low heat.

4 Remove the kebabs from the grill or barbecue when the vegetables are beginning to brown nicely and soften, and serve with the marinade or shoyu on the side. The kebabs can be served with brown rice and a green salad made from oriental leaves.

Plan 5

Breakfast choices
See page 82

Lunch choices
Choose one of the following:
- Chilled beetroot soup (see opposite)
- Bean salad with herbs (see page 102)
- A baked potato filled with Greek salad – feta cheese, tomato, onion, cucumber and black olives

Dinner choices
- Grilled/baked herring or mackerel served with seasonal vegetables and a squeeze of lemon juice
- Quinoa and wild rice pilaff (see page 103)

Desserts
Choose one of the following:
- Any kind of fresh fruit salad
- Organic yoghurt with fresh fruit

Snacks
- Any fresh fruit – melon, grapes, apple, pear, satsuma
- A fresh juice, smoothie or non-dairy milk shake
- Raw vegetable crudités with tahini, hummus or guacamole

Chilled beetroot soup (serves 2)

Ingredients

1 tsp olive oil
½ small onion, finely
  chopped
1 garlic clove, chopped
3 raw beetroot
½ tsp ground cumin

200–300g (7–10oz) canned
  chopped tomatoes
300ml (½ pint) water or
  vegetable stock
salt and black pepper
live yoghurt (optional)

1 Heat the oil in a saucepan, add the onion and garlic and cook gently for about 5 minutes until softened.

2 Prepare the beetroot: trim and peel them quickly, chop into slices, cut the slices into quarters and add to the pan. Cook for 5 minutes. Stir in the cumin and tomatoes with the liquid. Simmer until the beetroot is just tender, about 20 minutes. If the liquid looks as though it is going down rather fast, add a little more.

3 Blend the soup in a liquidizer and season to taste. Push the soup through a sieve with a wooden spoon into 2 bowls. Chill in the fridge for at least 2 hours. Serve with a swirl of live yoghurt, if wished, and some non-wheat bread.

Bean salad with herbs (serves 1)

Ingredients

20g (²/₃oz) dried haricot
  beans
20g (²/₃oz) dried black-eye
  beans
40g (1¹/₂oz) dried
  chickpeas
1 small red onion, chopped
6 olives, chopped
6 cherry tomatoes, chopped

salad leaves, e.g. rocket, flat-
  leaved parsley, coriander
handful of dandelion leaves

For the dressing:

1 tbsp lemon juice
2 tsp olive oil
¹/₂ tsp wholegrain mustard
¹/₂ tsp clear honey

1 Soak all the beans separately overnight; drain and
rinse. Put the haricots in a pan with fresh water. Bring to
the boil, then simmer gently. When they start to soften,
add the chickpeas and continue cooking until tender.

2 Boil the black-eye beans in water for 10 minutes in
another pan, then simmer until tender. Drain all the
cooked beans and rinse with fresh water.

3 Whisk the dressing ingredients and pour half over
the beans. Mix in the onion, olives and tomatoes.

4 Toss the salad leaves and dandelion greens in the
remaining dressing. Add the beans and serve at once.

Quinoa and wild rice pilaff (serves 1)

Ingredients

10g (1/3oz) wild rice
350–500ml (12–16fl oz)
   water
1 tsp rapeseed oil
1 small red onion, chopped
2 cardamom pods, crushed
a small pinch of cinnamon

black pepper
40g (1 1/2oz) quinoa
20 pine nuts
2 dried apricots, chopped
harissa or chilli sauce
   (optional)
mint leaves, to garnish

1 Put the wild rice in 150ml (1/4 pint) water, bring to the boil and simmer until cooked, about 40–50 minutes. Drain and set aside.

2 Warm the oil in a heavy pan with a lid, and add the onion. When it begins to soften, add the cardamom, cinnamon and black pepper. Add the quinoa and stir for 2–3 minutes. Add 200ml (7fl oz) water and bring to the boil, then cover and simmer for 10 minutes.

3 Add the pine nuts, check the liquid, adding more if necessary, and stir. Cook, covered, for 3 minutes, then check again and add the apricots. Stir in the cooked rice and cook, uncovered, until all the liquid has been absorbed. Check the seasoning, adding harissa or chilli sauce if liked. Serve, garnished with mint leaves. .

Plan 6

Breakfast choices
See page 82

Lunch choices
- Sweetcorn soup, served with non-wheat bread (see opposite)
- Kiwi and avocado salad (see page 106)

Dinner choices
- Your choice of organic oily fish, served with heaps of seasonal vegetables and a squeeze of lemon juice
- Roast vegetables with mash (see page 107), served with a crisp green salad and fish (optional)
- Two-egg wild mushroom omelette, served with choice of vegetables or salad

Dessert choices
Choose one of the following:
- Any kind of fresh fruit salad
- Blueberry salad (see page 95)

Snacks
- Any fresh fruit – melon, grapes, apple, pear, satsuma
- A fresh juice, smoothie or non-dairy milk shake
- Mixed nuts and seeds

Sweetcorn soup (serves 2)

Ingredients

1 medium onion, chopped
1 tsp olive oil
pinch of cayenne pepper
1 x 200g (7oz) can organic

sweetcorn, drained
600ml (1 pint) vegetable
   stock *or* water
salt and black pepper

1 Soften the onion in the olive oil gently in a large pan with a lid; don't let it burn but allow it to colour a little. When the onion is soft, add the cayenne pepper and stir thoroughly.

2 Add the sweetcorn and the vegetable stock or water. Cover and cook gently for 25 minutes – the liquid will reduce quite a lot.

3 Blend the soup thoroughly in a food processor or blender and check the consistency, adding another 100 ml (3½fl oz) liquid if wished. Reheat gently and then season to taste before serving.

Tip: If you like hot flavours, then a few flakes of dried red chilli can also be scattered on top as a garnish.

Kiwi and avocado salad (serves 1)

Ingredients

1 kiwi fruit, peeled

3 spring onions

1 ripe avocado

salad leaves

For the dressing:

squeeze of lime juice

1 tsp olive oil

a dab of honey

1 Slice the kiwi fruit and cut each slice into four. Finely chop the spring onions, and mix with the kiwi.

2 Make the dressing. Put the lime juice, olive oil and honey in a screwtop jar with lots of freshly ground black pepper. Seal the jar and shake it well, then taste, adding a little salt if wished. Pour over the kiwi and spring onions and leave for 30 minutes for the flavours to develop.

3 Cut the avocado in half and remove the stone; peel and then chop the flesh into chunks. Add these to the bowl containing the kiwi and spring onions, and stir very gently to coat the pieces in the dressing.

4 Arrange the salad leaves on a plate and arrange the kiwi, spring onion and avocado in the middle. Serve the salad immediately.

Roast vegetables with mash (serves 1)

Ingredients

1 x 200g (7oz) sweet potato
2 tsp olive oil
250g (8oz) chopped and
   peeled squash, centre
   and seeds removed
1 red onion, quartered

1 large fennel, sliced
1 red pepper, seeded and
   chopped
4 garlic cloves, unpeeled
1 large sprig of rosemary
juice of 1/2 orange

1 Preheat the oven to 200°C, Gas Mark 6. Bring a pan of water to the boil and drop in the whole, unpeeled sweet potato. Cook for 35–45 minutes until tender.

2 Put the olive oil in an ovenproof dish and pop it into the oven. When it is warm, add the squash, onion, fennel and red pepper. Tuck in the garlic and scatter rosemary leaves over the top. After 15 minutes, give the vegetables a stir, and return to the oven for 10 minutes. Season, stir again and roast for another few minutes.

3 Drain and peel the sweet potato, then mash with orange juice and black pepper. Remove the vegetables from the pan, fish out the garlic and squeeze the flesh out of the skin into the sweet potato; mash roughly. Serve with the roasted vegetables and a green salad.

Plan 7

Breakfast choices
See page 82

Lunch choices
- Carrot and lentil soup, served with non-wheat bread (see opposite)
- Tomato, onion and herb salad (see page 110)

Dinner choices
- Your choice of organic oily fish served with heaps of seasonal vegetables and a squeeze of lemon juice
- Masoor dhal with cauliflower (see page 111)
- Roast vegetables of your choice topped with crumbled feta cheese and herbs, served with hummus or guacamole and a crisp salad

Dessert choices
- Any kind of fresh fruit salad
- Orange and date salad (see page 91)

Snacks
- Any fresh fruit – melon, grapes, apple, pear, satsuma
- A fresh juice, smoothie or non-dairy milk shake
- Some raisins or other dried fruits

Carrot and lentil soup (Serves 2)

Ingredients

1 tsp olive oil
1 small red onion, chopped
200g (7oz) carrots,
    chopped
650ml (1 pint 2fl oz)
    vegetable stock or water

30g (1oz) green lentils,
    picked over and rinsed
juice of ½ small orange *or*
    1 mandarin
a few sprigs of fresh thyme
salt and black pepper

1 Warm the oil in a heavy pan, add the chopped red onion and cook gently, allowing it to brown a little, for 5 minutes. Add the carrots, stir well, and cook for 2 minutes before adding the stock or water and the lentils. Cook for 20 minutes and then add the orange or mandarin juice.

2 Remove the thyme leaves from the sprigs and drop them into the soup (reserve some for later). Cook for 5 minutes and add some black pepper. Remove from the heat, allow to cool a little and then blend, adding more liquid if you prefer a thinner soup. Reheat gently, check the seasoning and serve, garnished with the reserved thyme leaves.

Tomato, onion and herb salad (serves 1)

Ingredients

1 red onion, peeled and
  halved

3 medium tomatoes,
  seeded and chopped

1 tbsp olive oil

a large handful of coriander
  leaves

a large handful of
  flat-leaved parsley

salt and black pepper

1 Rinse the red onion in cold water, then soak for 10 minutes and chop coarsely – you need slightly less onion than tomatoes. Mix the chopped onion with the tomatoes in a large bowl, add the olive oil and a good grinding of black pepper, and stir well. Then cover the bowl with clingfilm and refrigerate for at least 1 hour.

2 Strip the leaves from the stems of the coriander and flat-leaved parsley, chop them roughly and add to the onion and tomato mixture. Stir well and add a little more olive oil if you like. Check the seasoning and serve immediately.

Tip: Prepare this salad in advance and then set aside to allow the flavours to mingle. Tomatoes sold on the vine often taste best.

Masoor dhal with cauliflower (serves 1)

Ingredients

1 tsp olive oil
1 small onion, chopped
1 garlic clove, chopped
1/4 tsp chilli powder
1/4 tsp ground cumin
1/4 tsp ground coriander
1/2 tsp turmeric
1/2 tsp paprika
50g (2oz) red lentils, rinsed

squeeze of lemon juice
1 small cauliflower, cut into
   medium-sized florets
water or vegetable stock
10g (1/3oz) desiccated
   coconut
10g (1/3oz) cashews
salt and black pepper
handful of mint leaves

1 Heat the oil in a heavy pan and cook the onion and garlic until they begin to brown. Add the chilli, cumin, coriander, turmeric and paprika and stir well. Stir in the lentils and lemon juice. Add the cauliflower florets, 150ml (1/4 pint) water or stock and the coconut.

2 Bring to the boil, then simmer, covered, for 10 minutes. Check that there is still some liquid left, adding more if necessary, and simmer for another 5 minutes.

3 Add the cashews and most of the mint. Simmer for 5 minutes, uncovered, until the liquid is absorbed. When the sauce is really thick, check the seasoning and serve garnished with the remaining mint leaves.

Plan 8

Breakfast choices
See page 82

Lunch choices:
- Avocado and tomato salad (see opposite)
- Crudités with Mexican dips (see page 114)
- Baked sweet potato with feta cheese, cherry tomatoes and salad leaves

Dinner choices
- Your choice of organic oily fish served with heaps of seasonal vegetables and a squeeze of lemon juice
- Vegetable fried rice with nori (see page 116)
- Pasta a picchi pacchi (see page 117)

Dessert choices
- Any kind of fresh fruit salad
- Blueberry salad (see page 95)

Snacks
- Any fresh fruit – melon, grapes, apple, pear, satsuma
- A fresh juice, smoothie or non-dairy milk shake
- Rice cakes, oatcakes or non-wheat bread with hummus, tahini, guacamole, goat's cheese, nut butter or honey

Avocado and tomato salad (serves 1)

Ingredients

1 large shallot *or* 2 smaller ones, peeled and finely chopped

2 tsp balsamic vinegar

3 medium tomatoes, sliced

1 ripe avocado

olive oil

salt and black pepper

1 Put the finely chopped shallot in a small bowl or container, such as an egg cup, with the balsamic vinegar while you prepare the salad.

2 Arrange the sliced tomatoes on one side of a plate. Cut the avocado into halves and remove the stone; cut through the flesh to the skin but not through the skin itself. Starting at the pointed end, peel the skin away with your fingers; if the avocado is ripe enough, this should be easy. Arrange the avocado slices on the other half of the plate.

3 Carefully, using a teaspoon, arrange the chopped shallot in a fine line between the two halves, leaving any excess vinegar behind. Drizzle olive oil over the salad, grind some black pepper over everything and put a little salt on the tomatoes. Serve immediately.

Crudités with Mexican dips (serves 2)

Ingredients

Use some of the following:
   spring onions; carrots,
   peppers and cucumber;
   celery sticks; chicory, cos
   and radicchio; cherry
   tomatoes; mushrooms;
   cauliflower florets

Red chilli bean dip:

50g (2oz) dried kidney
   beans
100g (3½oz) canned
   chopped tomatoes

1 garlic clove, chopped
pinch of chilli powder
squeeze of lemon juice

Guacamole:

1 ripe avocado, peeled and
   stoned
2 spring onions, chopped
1 red chilli, chopped
1 small tomato, seeded and
   finely chopped
squeeze of lemon juice
1 garlic clove, crushed

1 To make the red chilli bean dip: soak the beans overnight, then drain, rinse and put them in a pan. Cover with fresh water and boil for 15 minutes. Drain again and transfer to a clean pan. Add the tomatoes, garlic and chilli powder and simmer gently until the beans are soft, about 20 minutes. If they stick, add more liquid. Cool slightly, then blend to a paste. Add the lemon juice and blend again. Decant into a serving bowl and allow to cool completely. Before serving, grind black pepper over the top.

2 To make the guacamole: mash the avocado flesh roughly with a fork. Add the rest of the ingredients and mash well; check the taste and add a little black pepper. Decant into a serving bowl. If you need to store this dip, cover it and place in the fridge – letting the avocado stone sit in it during storage is supposed to stop it discolouring, but if you only keep it a short while and cover it well this should not be a problem.

3 Serve the dips surrounded by a selection of raw vegetable crudités.

SALSA

Ingredients

6 ripe plum tomatoes
½ red onion, finely
  chopped
1 red chilli, chopped

a handful of fresh basil
  leaves, torn
splash of olive oil and
balsamic vinegar

1 To make the salsa: dip the tomatoes briefly in boiling water – the skins should split, making it easier to peel them. Squeeze out the seeds and chop the flesh, then put in a serving bowl. Stir in the red onion and basil.

2 Pour a little olive oil and balsamic vinegar over the top. Leave for several hours to let the flavours develop.

Vegetable fried rice with nori (serves 1)

Ingredients

60g (2oz) brown rice, rinsed

½ sheet of nori

1 tbsp rice vinegar

1 tbsp shoyu

½ tsp sesame oil

½ tsp grated root ginger

2 tsp rapeseed oil

5 spring onions, chopped

1 carrot, cut into strips

½ green pepper, seeded and cut into fine strips

1cm (½in) root ginger, peeled and chopped

1 garlic clove, chopped

1 tsp sesame seeds

salt and black pepper

1 Cover the rice with cold water and bring to the boil. Cover the pan and simmer for 20 minutes, or until it is done but retains a bit of bite. Rinse thoroughly.

2 Toast the nori until it changes colour and gets crisp. Crumble into a dish. Whisk the vinegar, shoyu, sesame oil and ginger, and set aside.

3 Heat 1 teaspoon rapeseed oil and fry the spring onions, carrot and green pepper for 5 minutes. Add the ginger and garlic and cook, stirring, for 2–3 minutes. Stir in the remaining oil, sesame seeds and rice. Stir continuously until heated through and add half the sauce. Season and serve immediately, with the toasted nori on top and the remaining sauce on the side.

Pasta a picchi pacchi (serves 1)

Ingredients

250g (8oz) fresh plum
    tomatoes, peeled and
    chopped
1 tbsp olive oil
15g (½oz) blanched
    almonds, crushed
1 garlic clove, crushed

a handful of fresh basil,
    pounded with a mortar
    and pestle
small pinch of chopped
    chilli (optional)
75g (3oz) wheat-free
    spaghetti

1 Put all the ingredients except the spaghetti in a bowl. Cover and leave for 1 hour at room temperature.

2 Cook the spaghetti in a large pan of boiling water for about 6–8 minutes, or according to the packet instructions. Drain and serve with the raw sauce.

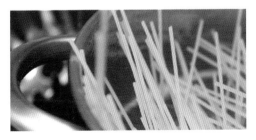

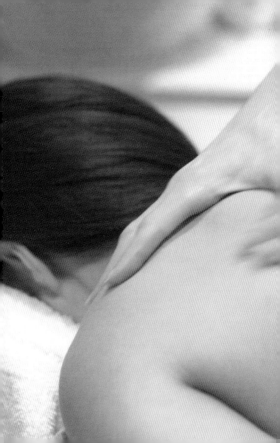

PART 5

Detox aids and therapies

It is important to eat well when detoxing but this is not the whole story. There are many other techniques that can support and intensify your efforts, helping you shed more toxins and cleanse your whole system. You can try some treatments yourself, in your own home, using easy-to-find products. Holistic therapies can also help you shed more of your toxin load. Some are extremely enjoyable, whereas others are decidedly not. The facts are here and it's up to you to find out what you're letting yourself in for.

SUPPLEMENTING YOUR DIET

Some of the treatments described in this chapter should be regarded as an essential part of your detox strategy, whereas others are an optional complement to it. You can choose the treatments that address your specific symptoms, or just the ones that appeal to you.

VITAMIN AND MINERAL SUPPLEMENTS

You should not need to take any vitamin and mineral supplements if you are eating a really varied diet with plenty of fresh fruits and vegetables of different colours, and lots of pulses, grains, nuts and seeds, but in practice, even if you follow the dietary guidelines earlier in this book (see page 46), it can be quite tricky covering all your basics.

Selenium

Intensive farming has significantly decreased the levels of vital minerals in our foods over the last 30 years. It is estimated that the average person's daily intake of selenium was 60 micrograms in 1974 and is now only half of that. Selenium is an essential nutrient for helping your liver to detoxify carcinogenic chemicals. Make sure your daily supplement contains 100–200mcg.

Multivitamins

Most detox diets recommend that you take a good multivitamin and mineral supplement, which contains at least 100 per cent of the recommended daily allowance (RDA) of vitamins A to E, plus the minerals calcium, iron, zinc, magnesium, potassium and selenium.

Choose a well-known brand but do read the label to watch out for any hidden ingredients, such as peanut oil, milk, gelatine, gluten, yeast or artificial flavouring and colours. Effervescent vitamins are best avoided because they can rot your teeth.

Essential fatty acids

The other supplement you are strongly recommended to take on a detox programme is an essential fatty acid blend with omega-3 (linolenic acid) and omega-6 (linoleic acid). Essential fatty acids (EFAs) are found naturally in nuts, seeds, green leafy vegetables, whole grains and oily fish, but it is estimated that eight out of

Taking supplements

Supplements should normally be taken after a meal and washed down with water. Don't take them with tea or coffee, as this could interfere with their absorption. If it's a one-a-day supplement, take it after the evening meal rather than breakfast, so it can do its work during the night when a lot of repair processes take place in the body.

ten people do not get enough from their diet. EFAs are essential for the production of prostaglandins that balance metabolic reactions, and imbalances can cause a range of symptoms, such as skin rashes, frequent thirst, dry hair and skin, low sex drive and a lowered immunity to infections. Take 500–1000mg evening primrose oil, 1–4g fish oil supplement or a dessertspoon of flaxseed oil. Udo's oil, available from health food shops and complementary chemists, is a good mix.

HERBAL SUPPLEMENTS

Made from the roots, stems, leaves, flowers, sap, bark, fruit and seeds of different plants, herbal supplements can be powerful detox helpers, stimulating liver and kidney function and protecting your organs and tissues from released toxins. Herbalists prefer to use tinctures made by soaking the herbs in an alcohol base, but you may find it more convenient to take tablets or capsules, made from dried or powdered extracts of the active component of the herb. You can also drink teas prepared from dried herbs, although the dosage will not be exact in this instance.

When buying herbs, look out for 'standardized' extracts which tell you how much of the active ingredient is present in each dose. Many cheap, non-standardized preparations contain very little. It's not advisable to take more than one herb at a time except under the supervision of a qualified herbalist, as there may be interactions (although you can drink herbal teas safely). Don't take herbs at all, without discussing it first with your doctor or specialist, if you are on any prescribed medication or have a chronic illness or health condition. For information on finding a herbalist or buying herbs by mail order, see page 182. Below is a selection of the best detox herbal supplements, their uses and doses.

Echinacea

If you are prone to colds or the flu virus, then try this immune system booster as part of your detox plan. Studies have shown that people taking echinacea get half as many infections as those who don't, and the ones they get tend to be less severe. It promotes sweating and can help with chronic fatigue syndrome following a viral infection. Take a 500mg tablet or 20 drops of tincture a day during a detox to help with cleansing. If you do get a cold or flu, take 300mg three times a day to help fight it off.

Milk thistle

The most famous detox herb, and rightly so. More than 300 studies have now shown that its active ingredient, silymarin, can protect liver cells from the poisonous effects of alcohol and other toxic chemicals. It inhibits free radical formation and boosts glutathione levels in the liver by over 33 per cent. It prevents poisons from penetrating the liver cells and also stimulates them to

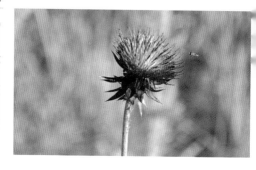

regenerate after cell damage. If you are not taking any other detox herbs to treat specific symptoms, choose this detox aid. Start with a dose of 100mg three times a day, standardized to at least 70 per cent silymarin, or take 20 drops of milk thistle tincture in water.

Artichoke extract

Globe artichoke is related to milk thistle. Studies have shown that artichoke leaf extracts reduce the effects of excess alcohol, lower cholesterol, increase bile secretion and improve digestive symptoms, such as bloating and flatulence. In a study of 550 people taking artichoke extracts for 66 weeks, abdominal pain was reduced by 76 per cent, constipation by 71 per cent and bloating by 66 per cent. If you experience a lot of digestive system problems, you should try taking standardized 320mg capsules one to three times a day with food.

Buchu

The leaves of this aromatic herb are diuretic and stimulate kidney cells to flush out toxins more quickly. Buchu has antibacterial properties that combat urinary tract infections and it helps prevent kidney stones. You can buy buchu leaves to make a tea from most health food shops, or ready-made teabags. Try buchu tincture if you don't urinate very often or you have a history of urinary tract infections, to make sure that your kidneys function effectively during a detox.

Dandelion

If you have a sluggish digestion and are prone to constipation, this should be your detox aid of choice. It stimulates the liver to increase the flow of bile and has a gentle laxative action. It is also good for addressing

Laxatives

Avoid buying strong laxatives, such as senna or dock, or mixtures containing them, if you suffer from constipation. The results may be rapid but the resultant speed of bowel movements can cause you to lose important nutrients and it is possible to become so dependent on laxatives that you are unable to have a normal bowel movement without them. Increase your fibre intake as a first course of action, then try dandelion tea; if this doesn't work, take aloe vera juice. Experiment until you find the combination that helps you pass the stools test on page 22.

hormone imbalances that are caused by oestrogen dominance, with symptoms such as cyclical breast pain in women. Drink three cups of dandelion tea or coffee a day or buy standardized 500mg extracts or tincture.

Ashwaganda

This is the supplement for a high-stress lifestyle. Studies suggest that it prevents the depletion of vitamin C and cortisol during periods of stress, reduces anxiety and promotes refreshing sleep. It boosts immunity and energy levels and can act as an aphrodisiac. Take two 250mg capsules a day or mix dried root powder with some boiling water and honey. .

Schisandra

If you have to take prescription drugs, work with toxic chemicals or have a problem with alcohol abuse, this can protect the liver and speed toxin removal from the body. The berries are the detoxification agent and can

Aloe vera gel

This can be helpful for treating skin conditions, e.g. eczema, psoriasis and sunburn, as it soothes and stimulates tissue regeneration in the area. In one study of 60 adults with psoriasis, those using aloe vera gel found that 80 per cent of rashes healed while only eight per cent noticed an improvement in the placebo group. Try it if you have reactive skin, but stop if it feels as though it is irritating it.

be taken either as a tea or in extracts of 300mg. It might even be worth taking schisandra preventively before painting your house or adding fertilizer to the garden, to raise your resistance to the toxins you'll be exposed to. (See page 169 for some healthier alternatives to common household products.)

Panax ginseng

For those people with a history of smoking, heavy drinking or taking street, OTC or prescription drugs, ginseng can be used to protect the body from cancers and reduce the damage caused by long-term exposure to the toxins in these substances. Don't take it if you have high blood pressure. You are advised to take ginseng for two weeks on, two weeks off. Choose a standardized product with no less than five per cent ginsenosides and start with around 600mg a day. Alternatively, boil 1 teaspoon of dried root for 10–20 minutes to make a tea, or take 20 drops root tincture.

Aloe vera

Fresh aloe vera juice, found in good health food shops, is a powerful tool for rectifying intestinal problems like bloating, flatulence, constipation and irritable bowel syndrome. Start with a small (50ml) daily dose or follow the guidelines on the product. Some people find the laxative effect of pure juice too powerful. You can also buy aloe vera tablets; one brand is sold under the label 'Colon Cleanse'.

EXERCISING DURING A DETOX

Moderate-intensity exercise will boost your detox on different levels. Opt for a mixture of aerobic exercise, a heart/lung workout that leaves you out of breath, and anaerobic exercise, designed to build muscle strength.

TOP 10 REASONS TO EXERCISE

1 Most people only breathe from the top third of their lungs, meaning that stale air and waste carbon dioxide stagnate lower down. Exercise that stimulates you to breathe deeply, using the whole of your lung capacity, clears out waste gases and lets more oxygen cross into your bloodstream. If you don't feel out of breath during aerobic exercise, you're not working hard enough.

2 Aerobic exercise makes your heart beat faster, pumping oxygenated blood round your system and through your liver and kidneys. Your cells are cleansed of waste materials and supplied with nutrients.

3 Both aerobic and anaerobic exercises get your lymphatic system moving, taking white blood cells to sites where they are needed and filtering out toxins from the tissues, thus helping to shift cellulite.

4 Exercise burns fat, releasing stored toxins into the bloodstream where they can be excreted through the liver, kidneys, lungs or skin.

5 Exercise that increases the amount you sweat will

help you to release toxins through the skin, including heavy metals, pesticides and pollutants.

6 Exercise stimulates the immune system to produce more disease-fighting cells. In a study of 150 people, those who walked on a regular basis contracted about half the number of colds as those who didn't.

7 Exercise can stimulate bowel movements as the movement of the outer, voluntary muscles provokes contraction of the inner, involuntary ones.

8 Exercise is a powerful mood enhancer and de-stresser, causing the brain to release feel-good chemicals, burning off stress hormones, lowering blood pressure and promoting restful sleep.

9 From our mid-30s onwards, hormonal changes cause us to lose muscle mass and store more fat, unless we combat this with exercise. When you lose muscle, you burn fewer calories and put on weight even if you eat the same amount of food. More weight equals more toxins. With regular strength-training exercise, you can keep the muscles you had and replace lost muscle.

Are you walking briskly?

Dawdling along the high street window-shopping and daydreaming does not count as exercise. If you want walking to be one of your daily detox exercises, you need to walk briskly, rolling from the heel through the foot and pushing off with the toes. Wear flat shoes with flexible soles that allow you to do this.

WHAT KIND OF EXERCISE?

The best exercise for you is the one that you enjoy the most and which fits in best with your lifestyle. Do an aerobic session one day, an anaerobic one the next.

• Aerobic exercises include tennis, football and ball sports; running and fast walking; skipping, trampolining, dance classes, swimming, cycling, skiing, skating and aerobic exercise classes (such as step or spinning).

• Anaerobic exercises include weight training in a gym, either on the equipment or with free weights; stretching; all kinds of yoga, and Pilates.

Important: Do not launch into an extreme exercise programme when you are detoxing; it will direct the blood to your muscles rather than to your detoxification organs, making you feel quite unwell.

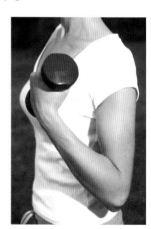

DAILY BATHING ROUTINE

Dry skin brushing feels fantastic, sloughing off all the dead skin cells and toxins excreted in sweat, as well as stimulating the lymphatic system and circulation. Go out and buy a soft, natural-bristle skin brush and use it once a day before you shower or bathe.

DRY SKIN BRUSHING

It is important when dry skin brushing to avoid any areas with broken skin as you work. The whole routine should take you around five minutes.

1 First of all, undress completely. Sitting on the edge of the bath, start brushing the sole of your left foot, then the left leg from your foot to the knee, with long, firm strokes.

2 When you have finished the lower leg, stand up and brush from the knee to the top of the thigh and over the buttocks. Repeat with your right leg.

3 Next brush your left arm from the palm of the hand up to the wrist, and then up to the shoulder. Repeat with the right arm.

4 Now brush your stomach, using gentle clockwise movements, then brush your back from the bottom up, and then the top down.

5 Don't brush your face – instead, just rub it with a dry, clean flannel.

SHOWERING OR BATHING

When you have finished skin brushing, have a shower or bath, using salts, seaweed or oils (see below). Make the water as hot as you can to create perspiration, and finish with a cool shower to increase the circulation and invigorate the lymphatic system. One minute under a cool shower or splashing yourself with cold water will make a big difference, so don't be a wimp about it.

Bath salts

Mineral salts encourage perspiration when added to a bath or used as an exfoliant scrub. Choose from Epsom salts, Dead Sea salts, Celtic Sea salts, or any other kind of marine salt you can find – but not ordinary table salt. Dissolve the salts in the warm bath water, then lie back and relax for at least five minutes before using a loofah or a brush to scrub away all the perspiration that the salts have drawn out. Alternatively, you can make a salt scrub by mixing your mineral salt with some olive oil and your choice of aromatherapy oil (see opposite).

Seaweed baths

Seaweed contains large quantities of minerals, such as calcium, phosphorus, magnesium, iron, iodine and sodium, as well as acids that can draw toxins through the pores of the skin. Therapeutic seaweed is available either in dried or powdered form from chemists. Steep it in the bathwater in a muslin bag or an infusion ball.

Alternatively, apply a seaweed gel all over your body before a bath. It's cheaper than the seaweed wraps you are offered in fancy spas, but often just as effective.

Aromatherapy oils

The essential oils from aromatic plants have many therapeutic properties. Some are ideal for intensifying a detox programme and/or dealing with many detox side effects, such as headaches and fatigue.

There are several ways to use these aromatic oils – in an aromatherapy burner, in a compress, for a massage, or to inhale in steam from a bowl of hot water – but one of the easiest is to add 5–10 drops of essential oil to a warm bath. Don't apply oils neat to the skin; always mix them with a carrier oil such as sweet almond, sunflower or apricot kernel oil (about 10 drops essential oil to 2 tablespoons carrier oil).

Detoxing oils

• To encourage the body to detox: juniper, lavender, geranium and rosemary.
• To relieve headaches: rosemary, peppermint and lavender.
• To help relieve stress: geranium, sandalwood, rose or ylang-ylang.
• To stimulate circulation: cypress, juniper, thyme or rose.
• For insomnia: clary-sage, camphor, Roman chamomile, lavender, rose, sandalwood or ylang-ylang.

OTHER DETOX AIDS

You now have all the essential elements for a basic detox programme, but you can speed up the process even more with detox aids, such as flower essences, foot patches and special detox kits.

FLOWER ESSENCES

Flower remedies are the concentrated essence of particular flowers which are dissolved in an alcohol base. They are designed to help with specific mental states, especially negative emotions, and the theory is that if you heal the mind, the body will follow.

Deciding which flower remedy to take depends on analysing your own mental state or getting a therapist who specializes in flower essences to do it for you.

Taking flower essences

You take flower essences by dotting them on to your pulse points four to six times a day, dotting them on your tongue, or by drinking a few drops in a glass of water. The amount of alcohol that you will ingest in this way is tiny, but if you want to be completely alcohol free during your detox, then it is best to stick with the pulse method. For information and advice on flower remedies and which to use, see opposite.

Types of essence

Many pharmacies and health stores stock a wide range of flower essences, and it is very important to choose the right one for you.

- Bush Flower Essences Purifying Essence is specifically designed for detoxing, both physically and emotionally. It should help you to let go of emotional baggage and leave you relieved and cleansed. Its exotic-sounding ingredients are Bush Iris, Bottlebrush, Dagger Hakea, Dog Rose and Wild Potato Bush.
- Bush Flowers Mountain Devil is also very good for detoxification and deep cleansing of the system, particularly if you are feeling angry and irritable.
- Bach Flowers Rescue Remedy is an excellent handbag standby to relieve headaches and problems with concentration or grogginess.
- Bach Flowers Crab Apple is also a cleansing remedy for those who feel unclean or polluted, physically or emotionally.
- Yarrow flower essence is said to detoxify and strengthen the body.

Flower remedies

- For more information and advice on all flower remedies, log on to: http://flowervr.com/
- To buy the flower remedies by mail order, you can either call Flower Essence Repertoire (01428 741672) or ring Nelson's Pharmacy (020 7495 2404).

FOOT PATCHES

According to Chinese medicine, the body has over 360 acupuncture points with more than 60 on the soles of the feet. Foot patches containing a blend of mineral and clay powders draw out toxins through the soles of the feet, taking the pressure off your liver, kidneys and other detox organs. They help release blockages in the lymphatic system, clear nerve pathways and accelerate toxin release in the blood.

Before you go to sleep, tape a white detox pad to the soles of your feet. You may feel a slight burning. In the morning, the pads will be brown and sticky with toxins. Claims made for the foot patches include improving blood circulation, increasing metabolism, relieving joint pain, stress and tension, and removing toxins.

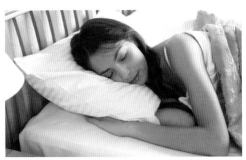

DETOX KITS

These may contain supplements to take during the first and second halves of a detox, so there is a 'cleansing' and then a 'restoring' phase. Typical cleansing supplements will contain milk thistle, dandelion, burdock root, kelp powder and psyllium. The restoration supplements will include lactobacillus or other probiotics, beetroot juice, and milk thistle. There is nothing wrong with using a detox kit if you are in good health and not taking other medications, but the levels of active ingredients you consume may not be as high as buying individual herbs.

WHAT SHOULD YOU TAKE?

Are you confused about what to do and take? There are many aids and therapies but the essential rules are:

- Only eat detox foods.
- Drink 2 litres (3^1/$_2$ pints) of water a day and as many herb teas as you like.
- Take a good multivitamin and mineral supplement, plus an essential fatty acid supplement.
- Take milk thistle or a herb to suit your symptoms.
- Exercise for at least 20 minutes a day.
- Dry brush your skin once a day before bathing.
- Foot patches, aromatherapy oils and flower essences are optional. Try them and see what you think works.
- In the following pages are spa treatments offered to help detox efforts – once again, the choice is yours.

CHOOSING A THERAPY

Most of the following therapies should only be carried out by a trained professional. Don't ever try them by yourself at home, and avoid them if you have any kind of medical condition, or if you are pregnant, unless you are specifically referred by your doctor.

CHELATION

Some alternative practitioners recommend this process for those people who have a build-up of heavy metals in their blood and tissues. Chelation is only performed in specialist clinics, where an intravenous drip is used to deliver 'chelating agents' which bind heavy metals, such as nickel, lead, mercury, cadmium and arsenic, and then pull them out through the stools, sweat and urine.

Uses and treatments

Chelating agents were first used during World War I to counteract the arsenic-based poison gas used in the trenches. They have also been used to treat people who are suffering from exposure to lead-based paints, or who have been contaminated with radioactivity. A clinical trial is taking place to examine chelation's effectiveness in treating atherosclerosis (narrowing of the arteries due to the build-up of cholesterol and other substances), but this will not report until 2008.

Should you try chelation?

Chelation is quite an extreme treatment and should be approached with great care. Check the qualifications of any clinic or practitioner offering it. You won't currently be referred for chelation on the NHS in the UK, but the British Heart Foundation is keeping an open mind on its possible benefits in the treatment of heart disease.

If you go to a clinic for chelation therapy to treat heavy metal toxicity, you will need between 10 and 40 sessions, depending on the level of toxins they detect in your initial tests. An intravenous drip will be put in your arm, containing vitamins, minerals and a chelating agent, and you will be told to lie back. Magnesium-based drips take between one and four hours but new calcium drips take just 15 minutes per session. You may feel tired and/or dizzy afterwards as your blood pressure may drop, so arrange for someone to pick you up from the clinic rather than trying to drive yourself home. Of course, this therapy will work out to be quite expensive, given the length of time it takes, the number of sessions, and the experienced medical supervision you will need to receive.

Colonic irrigation

In use since ancient Egyptian times, colonic irrigation is an effective method of getting rid of waste from a clogged-up colon by washing it out with water. Here's what happens at a session.

Finding a therapist

It should be relatively easy to find a colonic irrigation therapist, as most complementary health clinics will offer this service. To be registered to practise in the UK, a therapist must have trained in anatomy and physiology plus a body-based therapy, and they must also have taken a course at an approved hydrotherapy training school. Check before you get on the treatment table!

Treatment

A trained therapist will go over your medical history first and ask you to change into a gown. You then lie on your side with your knees up and a speculum connected to sterile rubber tubing is inserted into your rectum. You lie on your back with your knees bent and the water is turned on. You are asked to hold it in for as long as it feels comfortable, then the therapist releases the pressure, allowing the water and accumulated waste to flow away. The therapist will massage your lower abdomen to help with the elimination process. The flushing is repeated until the water runs clear, or until the therapist feels that you have had enough. At the first session, you might release waste equivalent to 20–30 bowel movements, as the entire 2-metre (6-ft) length of the colon is cleansed.

From the waste evacuated, the therapist should be able to advise you on modifications to your diet which will improve your digestion. They will say, for example, if you need to eat more fibre or less fat or sugar. The first session will usually last 30–45 minutes and you may be advised to return at a later date for more treatments. After a session, you should take probiotic supplements to replace any intestinal bacteria washed away.

What are the effects?

Most people say that they feel distinctly healthier after colonic irrigation, and you may find that your weight has dropped by several pounds without those clogged-up waste materials. Your digestive system will function more effectively, as will the liver and kidneys. If you were prone to headaches before the treatment, you might find they clear up now, and many people claim to sleep better. However, the effects might not be particularly long-lasting.

Coffee enemas

Certain spas offer enema treatments, or you can buy your own enema kit in pharmacies or over the internet, but the coffee enema, generally used for detox purposes, is quite a harsh one. Coffee grounds irritate the muscles of the colon, encouraging it to contract and squeeze out its contents. The caffeine is quickly absorbed through the veins of the rectum and taken in the blood up to the liver where, it is claimed, it dilates the bile ducts, stimulating toxins to be passed into the intestine and thus expelled.

DETOXING HOLIDAYS

If you want to combine detoxing with a holiday, you can book into a spa resort that offers a complete detox package in idyllic surroundings. You might fast during the week, taking in only detox cocktails (psyllium husk and clay, for example), herbal laxatives and one daily bowl of vegetable broth. You will also be taught how to administer your own daily coffee enema and may even be encouraged to sift through the evacuated waste material to see what comes out. Guests at such detox resorts have described finding tapeworms, liver flukes, huge chunks of undigested meat, yellow fatty deposits and string-like shreds of various hues.

After a week of fasting, raw fruits and vegetables may be consumed for the next few days. Everyone loses weight and emerges with clear, glowing skin and improved digestion, but whether they keep the weight off will depend on the eating habits they maintain on

Spa holidays

At the following website, www.andalucia.com/health/alternative-health, you will find descriptions of over 50 different alternative therapies by health journalist Dee McMath, who has personally tried most of them. If you've ever wondered what Okkaido or Harmonic Resonance Therapy involve, here's your chance to find out.

their return from holiday. Certainly, sifting through your own waste materials can help to put you off eating unhealthily, but it is not to everyone's taste.

TRADITIONAL CHINESE MEDICINE

Chinese therapists see good health as a harmonious balance in the body between the forces of yin and yang, with energy known as chi flowing freely along meridians. If chi becomes blocked or imbalanced, illness can result. In Chinese medicine, detoxification involves removing 'devil toxins', which include heat, cold, parasites, damp, fire and food toxins.

Diagnosis and treatment

At an initial consultation, the therapist will look at your general appearance, examine your tongue, ask about your lifestyle and medical history, and take your pulses from three positions on each wrist. Depending on the diagnosis, they may treat you with acupuncture – thin needles are inserted at acupoints along the meridians to free blockages and stimulate the flow of *chi*. You may be offered herbal detoxification formulas to boost the metabolism to burn fats and clean up the digestive system. These remedies could be herbs for brewing tea, or pills, powders or pastes. Some therapists use a mix of acupuncture and herbs, as required. There will usually be follow-up sessions to chart progress and adjust the treatments according to how the body is responding.

What can it treat?

Traditional Chinese Medicine (TCM) is especially recommended for treating digestive disorders, such as irritable bowel syndrome; chronic skin conditions like eczema; fatigue and depression; hormonal imbalances such as PMS; endometriosis and poor sperm count, and infertility (male and female). It can produce results with chronic conditions that Western methods fail to help.

Self-diagnosis and treatment of medical conditions are not recommended, but at some TCM centres you can describe your symptoms to the practitioner behind the counter and receive an appropriate remedy on the spot. TCM can be very successful for treating people undergoing withdrawal from drugs and alcohol.

Alcohol and drugs

Alcohol creates liver and gall bladder imbalances, which brings about a combination of excessive dampness and heat. Many drugs are processed

Auriculotherapy

In this form of Chinese acupuncture, little pins are inserted at the acupoints in the ear. It is a powerful method of treating addictions of all kinds, from drugs to alcohol to smoking. When a craving comes on, you twiddle the pin(s) to stimulate the appropriate acupoint, which reactivates the treatment and helps to stop you backsliding.

through the liver, making it heated and congested, so the liver blood becomes weak and deficient. TCM formulas focus on clearing and nourishing the liver and gall bladder, while at the same time treating the heart, to help calm the mind and nervous system.

AYURVEDIC DETOXIFICATION

Ayurveda is an ancient Indian system of healthcare and, like Traditional Chinese Medicine, it is based on the idea of balance within the body. There are three primary *doshas* – *kapha*, *pitta* and *vata* – of which we all have different degrees in our bodies and personalities. Treating the symptoms of unwellness will involve balancing these doshas.

Detoxification methods

Ayurveda is a complete holistic system which should only be followed under the supervision of a qualified practitioner. The main method of detoxification, which is called Panchakarma, works on several levels. First, your diet is cleared out and cleansing foods, such as kichari (made from basmati rice, mung beans and vegetables), are recommended. Herbal supplements are given to cleanse the bowel and flush out toxins from the liver, blood, sweat glands and skin. These will be designed according to your dosha balance. You may be given a massage with herbal oils, heat treatment to open the circulatory channels, and enemas.

Nasya

Otherwise known as nose cleansing, this is part of ayurvedic detoxing. It involves flushing a medicated oil through the nose and sinuses, in one nostril and out the other, to cleanse toxins from the head and neck. Results can be marked if you suffer from headaches and migraine, nasal allergies, sinusitis, poor memory or eyesight, and certain neurological conditions.

Benefits

Recent tests of ayurvedic detoxing at the University of Colorado found that those who had undergone several detoxes had significantly lower levels of PCBs, DDT and pesticide residues than the control group. It appeared to be particularly effective on fat-soluble toxins of the

The doshas

Our constitution is determined by the state of our parents' *doshas* at the moment we are conceived. We all have a balance of the three:

• *Vata* is the driving force, relating to energy and the nervous system.

• *Pitta* is fire, relating to metabolism, digestion, enzymes and bile.

• *Kapha* is related to water in the mucous membranes, phlegm, fat and lymphatic system.

A series of physical examinations and questions will enable ayurvedic practitioners to discern your dominant *doshas*.

kind associated with hormone disruption, suppression of the immune system, allergies, and diseases of the liver and skin. If there is a good ayurvedic clinic near you, it could be worth doing an ayurvedic detox. Some complementary chemists stock well-known ayurvedic remedies that they can recommend to treat individual symptoms, but a complete Panchakarma detox must be done under professional supervision.

DETOXIFYING MASSAGE TECHNIQUES

There are dozens of different kinds of massage, but the following can be used specifically to enhance the effects of a detox programme.

Manual lymphatic drainage

In the 1930s, Dr Emil Vodder created this technique in order to stimulate the lymphatic system and help it to eliminate toxins in the cells. MLD is an advanced massage therapy in which the therapist uses special rhythmic pumping techniques to move the skin in the direction of the flow of lymph back to the lymph nodes. It can be used to treat lymphedema (swelling due to fluid accumulation in the tissues), cellulite, sinusitis and arthritis, and it can help to encourage healing after surgery. It's a very pleasant type of massage treatment that would be a useful addition to any detox programme, although it may take several sessions before you see any positive results.

Hot stone therapy

This type of massage uses heated volcanic lava stones. Their heat helps to increase heart rate and stimulate circulation, helping to flush the muscles of toxic waste products. This therapy is also used to treat depression, stress, PMS, stiff joints and certain skin disorders.

Treatment

In one version of the treatment, you lie on the heated stones and are given a massage with aromatherapy oils. In yet another form of the therapy, the stones themselves are used to massage your arms, legs and back. Sometimes cold stones are used as well, to further stimulate the circulation. The treatment is very relaxing and promotes restful sleep.

Rolfing

This kind of deep tissue massage was developed by American biochemist Dr Ida P. Rolf in the 1930s. Practitioners are trained to feel for imbalances in the

Naturopathy

Naturopaths take a broad, holistic view of health and can recommend treatments across a number of different therapies. They will advise on diet, supplements and herbs, exercise and physical therapies, and they can also offer psychological support techniques such as counselling. To learn more, look at www.naturopathy.uk.com

quality, texture and temperature of tissues and thus determine how to reintegrate the body, 'bringing physical balance in the gravitational field'. Rolfing therapists work on your body, using their hands, fingers, knuckles and even elbows, and the experience can be uncomfortable at times, but it could be worth trying as part of your detox.

Shiatsu massage

The aim of Shiatsu massage is to balance the flow of *chi* energy along the meridians, and practitioners apply pressure to exactly the same acupoints that are used in acupuncture. Some people report a 'healing crisis' after treatments, such as a headache or flu-like symptoms that last up to 24 hours. These are seen as positive signs that toxins and pent-up emotions are being released. The number of follow-up sessions recommended will vary according to the toxicity of your system.

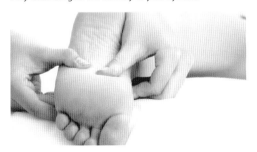

Swedish massage

Swedish massage therapists manipulate the muscles and tissues to stimulate the circulatory, nervous and digestive systems and ease stiffness. They believe that emotional tension from past traumas is stored within the muscles and part of their role is to try and release it. It has proved extremely effective at treating a range of stress-related conditions as well as depression, insomnia, digestive disorders and premenstrual syndrome.

Reiki

Reiki is a system of healing developed by the Japanese theologian Mikao Usui, in which the practitioner makes himself into a channel through which energy flows into the patient to heal their imbalances. You lie fully clothed while the therapist places his hands in a sequence of positions that cover the whole body. When detoxing, reiki can support and encourage positive personal change – improving your diet, getting more exercise and even reducing cravings for alcohol and tobacco.

OSTEOPATHY

Osteopathy is a manipulation therapy which reduces strain placed on the body from physical causes, such as bad posture or injury, and emotional causes, such as stress, anxiety and fear. It can help to relieve digestive disorders, including constipation, hormonal imbalances causing menstrual pain, headaches, insomnia and depression, among other things. If you tell an osteopath that you are detoxing, they can palpate your liver to stimulate its action and support its efforts.

Craniotherapy

Many osteopaths will also use craniosacral therapy, or craniotherapy techniques. The brain and spinal cord are surrounded by cerebrospinal fluid that flows with a steady rhythm when we are healthy. The osteopath is trained to detect any tiny variations in the movement of this fluid that indicate emotional or physical trauma in the bones, organs or areas of the body supplied by spinal nerves at each point.

Treatment

This is surprisingly relaxing and restful. While you lie on your back, the therapist places their fingers alongside your spine, moving up it, vertebra by vertebra, in order to feel for places where the flow is restricted, and they can then free it up just by using gentle pressure.

The effects of craniotherapy

Craniotherapy has a deeply relaxing effect on people and can improve the function of the immune, digestive, respiratory, hormonal and circulatory systems. Some people experience a healing crisis during the 24 hours after their treatment but it should not be too serious. This gentle therapy tends to be highly recommended by all who try it.

HYDROTHERAPY

This blanket term is now used to refer to all kinds of water-based treatments. In the following pages, you will find descriptions of the different hydrotherapy methods that can be particularly useful when you are on a detox programme. The choice is down to personal preference as they are all pleasant and effective.

The Kneipp Method

A nineteenth-century Bavarian monk, Father Sebastian Kneipp, invented this technique which claims to cure illness by helping the body to get rid of its waste products. It uses a programme of hot and cold baths, steam baths and herbal wraps to cleanse and detoxify, improve the circulation, stimulate the flow of lymph and help the digestive system.

Treatments

A therapist will talk to you first and will then design a programme to suit your specific problems, but the elements could include one or some of the following:

* A hot herbal bath with lavender and rosemary, and possibly some salts and oils as well.
* A moor bath, which is a hot, muddy sludge of herbs in which you relax for up to 20 minutes.
* High-powered jets of hot or cold water directed onto your back to stimulate the circulation.
* Sitz baths – one filled with hot water and one with

cold water, which are used as a circulation stimulator. You stand with your feet in the hot water until they are warmed through, then step into the cold water bath until they cool down, and repeat the process several times. Salts may be added to intensify the effects.

- A herbal wrap in which you lie with herbs bound tightly around you to make you sweat and draw out any impurities through the pores.
- These water-based sessions may be followed by a Swedish massage.

Thalassotherapy

This form of hydrotherapy is very popular at many spa resorts. The term is derived from the Greek word *thalassos*, meaning sea, and is used for any treatment involving seawater or seaweed. Seawater is rich in minerals, which are great for drawing out toxins, cleansing and toning the skin, so many thalassotherapy treatments involve swimming in a heated seawater pool or being pummelled with jets of seawater.

Oral hygiene

Keeping your mouth free of bacteria is extremely important. Bacteria tcan cause tooth decay, receding gums and even heart disease. Buy one of the new sonic toothbrushes that remove more plaque than manual ones, and floss and scrape your tongue as well as brushing your teeth. Visit a dental hygienist for a thorough clean.

Thalassotherapy is very relaxing, and most people will notice a great improvement in their skin texture and tone after just one of these enjoyable treatments.

Seaweed wraps

Seaweed wraps are a very popular technique, and are said to boost the circulation, stimulate the metabolism and encourage the elimination of toxins. They are particularly recommended for treating cellulite, sagging skin and stretch marks, and some people even claim to lose a few centimetres after a single wrap.

Finding therapists

To find a clinic offering the therapies described, check your local directory or surf the internet. Many complementary health clinics offer a wide range of treatments, and you can be cross-referred between therapists. To find a spa holiday, ask your travel agent or look on the net!

Treatment

Generally, a trained therapist will smoothe seaweed paste all over your body, targeting specific areas if you wish. You are wrapped in some warm thermal sheets and left for up to 45 minutes, after which you must shower it all off. It is important to drink extra water after a seaweed wrap to prevent dehydration.

SAUNAS AND STEAM BATHS

Many local gyms and health clubs now offer saunas (a hot dry room) or steam baths (hot and steamy) to help eliminate impurities through sweating. Don't be tempted to stay in and overdo it. Start with a five-minute sauna or steam bath, and don't spend more than 20 minutes in there or you could feel very dizzy and unwell. Some people use a spatula to scrape off sweat and released toxins. Alternatively, you can have a good rub-down with a loofah or brush in the shower afterwards to slough off dead skin cells as well as waste products. Do as the Swedes do and follow up with a stimulating cold shower afterwards.

Safety guidelines

Resist the temptation to keep throwing extra water on a sauna's coals to increase the heat. If you suffer from high blood pressure, heart disease, asthma or epilepsy, you should avoid saunas or steam baths, as they could exacerbate your condition.

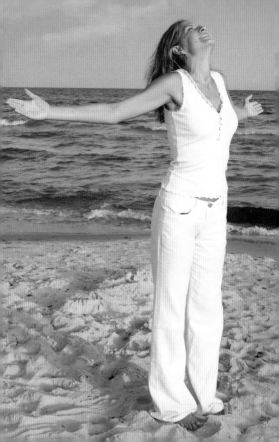

PART 6

Making it safe

We are surrounded by toxins. They could be in your toothpaste and antiperspirant, in the chair you are sitting on, the carpet below your feet, and the cleaning products, paints and varnishes you have used all over your home. In the garden, they are in the pesticides that stop slugs eating your plants and the creosote on the fence. You may not be able to do much about the toxins in the air you breathe – but for all the rest, there are safer alternatives.

EVERYDAY TOXINS

Beware! Reading this chapter and finding out about all the nasty substances in the products you use daily will almost certainly change your shopping habits forever!

PLAYING WITH CHEMISTRY

Twentieth-century chemists were extremely proud of themselves when they invented brand-new chemical compounds that could dissolve even the toughest dried-in grease in our ovens, make our laundry whiter-than-white, penetrate and plump out ageing skin cells, kill all known germs, and keep us odour-free all day long. Synthetic materials, like rayon and nylon, were all the rage, carpets were treated to make them virtually indestructible, and timber was sealed so that it would never rot. Alternatively, you could buy brand-new particleboard products made of wood fibre and held together with synthetic resin. Life was getting better and better for us all – or was it?

Animal testing

If you are against animal testing, you should be aware that when a label says a product is 'not tested on animals', it can simply mean that although the whole product was not tested on animals, several of the key ingredients may have been.

Cumulative effects

None of these products make you keel over gasping and wheezing on first exposure, but the toxins they contain have a cumulative effect with long-term exposure that scientists are still investigating today. They are only now finding out that cosmetics and personal care items containing parabens seem to be linked to breast cancer – although it is hardly surprising, since parabens mimic the action of oestrogen in the body. It was long thought that mercury could not leach out of fillings once they were in place, but autopsies are finding a direct correlation between the amount of mercury in the brain cells and the number of fillings that a person has in their teeth.

Dry-cleaning solvents containing perchloroethylene (perc, for short) are excellent at removing stains without damaging the fabric, but they have now been linked to cancer, liver and nervous system damage, infertility and hormone disruption.

What is 'natural'?

Maybe the time has come to cut the chemistry and just go back to nature in our quest for good health. But what exactly does 'natural' mean? The truth is that it is virtually meaningless when the word is used on a product label. By law, only a small percentage of the ingredients that are listed need to be 'natural' for this term to be used.

Check the packaging

You will find some confusing phrases used on product packaging. The term 'derived from natural coconut oil', for example, can actually refer to cocamide DEA, a foaming agent used in some shampoos, which is extracted from coconut oil by the addition of a solvent known as diethanolanine, which is widely thought to be carcinogenic.

What is 'organic'?

Can you trust the term 'organic'? Some manufacturers have played with the word in the past, for example claiming to use 'organic herbs' in a product that is otherwise entirely composed of synthetic chemicals. In theory, the unscrupulous could even claim that a toxic petrochemical preservative, such as methyl parabens, is organic, because it comes from leaves that rotted thousands of years ago to become crude

Alternatives to dry cleaning

Greenpeace believes that the best option currently available is wet cleaning, a process in which garments are immersed in water and eco-friendly detergents, then carefully dried and stretched back into shape. However, this will cause more fabric deterioration than dry cleaning. If you decide to dry clean a garment, hang it outdoors to air for as long as possible afterwards, so that the toxic residues can evaporate.

oil, which was then used to make this preservative. But, in fact, the organic market is controlled very carefully. Organic standards boards only grant organic status to those products that pass stringent testing procedures. To be on the safe side, look out for organic kitemarks and certification if a product claims to be organic. The companies recommended throughout this chapter are all trustworthy.

PERSONAL GROOMING

Toxins are eliminated through the skin via perspiration, but they can also be absorbed through the skin via hair follicles and sebaceous glands (although not through sweat glands). You will not ever hear any skincare manufacturers claiming that their products penetrate through the skin and into the blood circulation, because they would then be classified as drugs and subject to much more stringent testing and regulation. However, there is plenty of evidence that skin does absorb some ingredients from skincare preparations because they are turning up in our blood, urine, organs and tissues. Scientists often find phthalates in urine, parabens in breast tumours, and synthetic fragrances like musk xylene in human fat.

It is ironic that the big cosmetic companies pour so much research funding into the development of new products that help to disguise the signs of ageing (anti-wrinkle creams, hair-thickening shampoos and conditioners, firming body lotions) yet they use ingredients that some researchers suspect of being carcinogens, neurological toxins, immune suppressants and hormone disruptors, so the net effect can be drastically ageing!

Safety tests

In the US, the Environmental Working Group tested 120 different cosmetic products, including shampoos, moisturizers, foundations and lip balm, and found ingredients certified by the US Government as 'known or probable carcinogens' in each and every one. In 2005, the US Food and Drug Administration declared that consumers should be told that many commercial shampoos, deodorants, perfumes, nail polishes, hand creams, hair dyes and bubble baths have not been safety tested, despite the fact that they commonly contain chemicals that disrupt the hormones, are carcinogenic and disrupt the nervous system.

Deodorants

To avoid parabens and aluminium salts, opt for alum crystal deodorants. They don't block the sweat glands but they inhibit bacterial growth in your sweat, which is what causes the odour. They are available in spray, roll-on, cream or the original crystallized rock form from chemists or the organic websites listed at the end of the book.

Phthalates

These are solvents found in fragrance and nail polish, as well as a substance added to plastics to make them more flexible. They have been linked to liver and thyroid damage, cancer, low sperm counts in men, miscarriages and birth defects. They are not easy to avoid, however, because they will not be listed on the ingredients label.

Parabens

Parabens (methyl, propyl and butyl) have all been linked to breast cancer (which can affect men as well as women, although less commonly) and they can also cause contact skin rashes.

DEA-related compounds

Topical application of DEA-related compounds (such as cocamide, lauramide and myristamide) has been linked to cancer by some experts.

Ceteareth-12

An emulsifier called Ceteareth-12 may contain dangerous levels of the carcinogenic ethylene oxide and dioxane.

Antiperspirants

These often contain aluminium salts that prevent the body from sweating. Aluminium build-up in brain cells has been linked to Alzheimer's disease.

Skin irritants

Many cosmetic additives can be skin irritants, such as lanolin, glycerol and cetyl alcohol, which are found in a wide range of products.

Avoiding harmful chemicals

The best way to steer clear of harmful ingredients is to opt for organic brands of everything you apply to your skin, including body- and face-care products, makeup, soaps, sunscreen, toothpaste and all other toiletries. You should be able to find them in large chemists or department stores, or try the websites listed on page 184 (many will send you catalogues on request).

MERCURY FILLINGS

Most British adults have at least one or two mercury fillings in their mouths, yet research shows that the average-sized filling contains 750,000 micrograms of mercury and releases around 10 micrograms a day. This vapour is inhaled and travels up to the hippocampus of the brain, which controls memory. People with Alzheimer's disease have mercury levels in their brains

Allergy help

Allergy UK has a chemical sensitivity division with lots of handy tips and alternatives for those who are allergic to everyday products. For details, see page 182.

that are two to three times higher than those who do not. Low-level mercury exposure can damage the brain, heart, lungs, liver, kidneys, thyroid, pituitary, adrenal glands, immune system, and just about every aspect of body function.

Replacing fillings

Should you rush to have your mercury fillings replaced? Certainly not, say most experts. Removing fillings can generate much more mercury vapour as well as stray particles as your dentist drills into them with a high-speed drill. If you are worried that your fillings are damaging your health, find a specialist who will test your urine for heavy metal content. If your levels are high, seek out a dentist who specializes in amalgam removal and only have one or two fillings replaced at a time. A rubber dam should be used to prevent you swallowing any particles and a high-speed suction device should be in your mouth at all times. You may also be given a nose mask to stop you inhaling mercury vapour (if it is not offered, then ask for one).

Some experts recommend that you undergo chelation therapy after filling removal to rid your system of any ingested mercury. If you ask your dentist, they will probably recommend that it's safer to leave mercury fillings in than take them out. Obviously, if a filling breaks or falls out anyway, that is the time to replace it with a safer (and more attractive) white alternative.

HOUSEHOLD CLEANING PRODUCTS

In the US, 12 per cent of emergency calls to the Poison Control Center are due to people ingesting household cleaning products. The damage that they do if you accidentally swallow them is very clear, but it is less obvious what's happening when we inhale them or absorb ingredients through our skin. You will probably want to avoid any cleaning products that contain the following substances.

Chlorine bleaches

These are found in toilet cleaners, washing powders and dishwasher detergents, and they can create carcinogenic substances when broken down. If they come into contact with products containing ammonia, a gas called chloramine is formed that can cause severe respiratory reactions.

A cleaner home?

Over the past 20 years, our consumption of household cleaning products has risen sharply in the UK, and there is a corresponding rise in the level of VOCs (volatile organic compounds) in the atmosphere. These can cause irritation of the airways when present in low concentrations and, according to a 2003 study, may increase the risk of childhood asthma. So make sure that you use more eco-friendly and healthy alternatives.

Optical brighteners

These give the illusion of whiteness by attaching themselves to fabrics and reflecting bright light, but they can cause severe skin irritation.

Butyl cellulose

This is found in heavy-duty all-purpose cleaners and can be absorbed through the skin and lungs. Some experts think it causes liver and kidney damage. At low levels, it may be responsible for headaches, dizziness, nausea and fainting.

Anionic surfactants

These are present in some cleaners and they can be contaminated with carcinogenic nitrosamines.

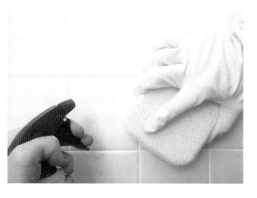

Carpet cleaners

These often contain butyl cellulose (see above) and may also contain perchloroethylene (the dry cleaning fluid, see page 159).

Phosphates

These are used in washing powder to improve cleaning and soften the water but they pollute our waterways by encouraging the growth of algae that starve the water of oxygen, killing fish and plant life.

Oven cleaners and metal polishes

Oven cleaners may contain 'lye', which gives off toxic fumes that can burn the skin and eyes. Metal polishes contain petroleum products that can damage the nervous system, kidneys and eyes.

Avoiding toxins

The list goes on! To try to avoid any toxic nasties, you should always choose a reputable organic brand in the supermarket (look for the certification logo), or buy your cleaning products from a reputable organic source (see page 184 for more information on companies and websites).

You might also want to consider using some of the old-fashioned natural cleansing solutions (see the suggestions opposite). These are often more effective than their modern chemical equivalents.

Natural cleaning

Here are some useful tips for cleaning in a more natural way in the time-honoured tradition. You may be surprised how well they work!

• Use vinegar in warm water to clean work surfaces, chrome, mirrors and glass.

• Polish the furniture with beeswax mixed with a little lemon essential oil.

• Freshen the air with your choice of aromatherapy oil in a sprayer full of water.

• Clean your oven with some bicarbonate of soda, hot water and stainless steel wool.

• Choose laundry soap instead of detergents and add half a cup of washing soda as a softener.

• Bleach white clothes in sunlight, or add some soda crystals to your wash.

• To descale your kettle, cover the element with equal quantities of vinegar and water, bring to the boil and then leave to soak overnight before scrubbing clean.

• To clean the toilet bowl, mix a paste of borax and lemon juice and leave for 20 minutes before scrubbing.

• For an effective cleaner for the bath, basin and tiles, just mix together baking soda, white vinegar, lemon essential oil and tea tree oil.

• To clean carpets or rugs, mix warm water, organic liquid soap, 1 tsp borax and a splash of vinegar. Sponge on, leave to dry and then vacuum off.

IN THE HOME

You have probably heard about the risks associated with paints, paint strippers, fuels, glues and permanent markers that contain volatile organic compounds (VOCs). The fumes from these can cause nausea, headaches and drowsiness, and prolonged exposure has been linked with cancer. Next time you redecorate your home, make sure that you choose organic, water-based paints, stains, sealants, thinners and markers, which emit only natural, pleasant fragrances.

Carpets

Many carpets are treated with pesticides, fungicides and dyes that can give off vapours that we inhale or chemicals that can be absorbed through the skin. The latex backing used on 95 per cent of carpets contains

Sanitary protection

Nearly all the major-brand tampons contain a mixture of rayon, which creates an ideal environment for the staphylococcus bacteria that causes toxic shock syndrome, as well as conventionally grown cotton, which has been exposed to many kinds of pesticides and fertilizers. Some of the chemicals used to bleach tampons have been implicated in the formation of dioxin, which can harm the inside of the vagina and may be linked to endometriosis. Choose organic tampons or pads.

styrene, a suspected carcinogen, and carpets can also contain volatile organic compounds and formaldehyde, low levels of which can irritate the eyes, nose and throat. The adhesive used for office carpets, known as 4-phenylcyclohexene (4-PC), is thought to contribute to 'sick building syndrome'. The healthiest carpets are hessian-backed and not treated with pesticides; choose organic wool cotton or hemp without biocides (to deter mould) or stain protectors.

Cushions

Watch out for polyurethane stuffing in sofa cushions, as some experts think it can give off toxic chemicals we inhale while watching TV. Ideally, use cushions stuffed with cotton or wool, but polyester fill is next best.

Woods

Synthetic urea formaldehyde resin is often used in manufactured woods (such as MDF, particleboard or chipboard). However, fumes continue to leak from these products for years, so it is best that you avoid manufactured woods. Some timber treatments can also be toxic, containing lindane (now banned, but could be found on older wood products and is linked to breast cancer), PCP (an organochlorine fungicide) and other insecticides and colourings. Always opt instead for organic wood which has been treated with natural chemicals including beeswax and borax.

Fabrics

We spend hours every night surrounded by bed linen; during the day, our skin is in constant contact with our clothes, so it makes sense to think about the chemicals used in making fabrics. Synthetic fabrics, e.g. nylon and rayon, are produced using a wide range of chemicals; more than 35 herbicides and pesticides are used to grow conventional cotton crops. To avoid these chemicals, you should opt instead for organic cotton or hemp. All the dyes used are plant or mineral based, and no heavy metals or harmful chemicals are used in the dyeing or finishing processes.

Fires

Get all your oil or gas fires checked out regularly by a qualified engineer to ensure they are functioning correctly and are not slowly poisoning you when in use. Although it is less common now, you still hear of people dying in their sleep while a faulty heater pumped out carbon monoxide into the atmosphere.

Mattresses

The wool used to stuff mattresses may be chemically treated, and research shows that these chemicals can emit vapours we breathe in as we sleep. Cover your mattress with a cotton barrier cloth or buy a new, organic one. You should avoid plastic sheets (such as those used when children are being potty-trained), as the plastic can give off harmful emissions.

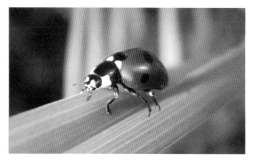

INSECTICIDES

None of us want our homes overrun by ants, clothes eaten by moths or barbecues ruined by a plague of mosquitoes, but any sprays or powders that cause insects to drop dead can't do us much good either.

Non-toxic bug control

Fortunately, there are plenty of natural, non-toxic ways of dealing with common bugs in the home and garden. Try the following and see for yourself.

- The herb tansy, planted in the garden, will deter ants. Indoors, pile some dried mint, chilli powder or borax at strategic points.
- Finely ground eggshells will deter slugs in the garden, around your vegetables and favourite plants, and act as a fertilizer as well.

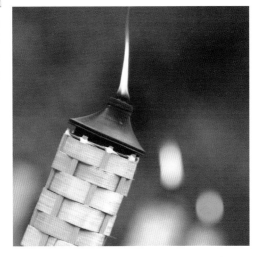

Headlice

If your child comes home from school with headlice, do not buy over-the-counter treatments containing malathione, a strong chemical that is rapidly absorbed into the tissues. Blend lavender, tea tree and eucalyptus oils in warmed olive oil and apply all over the hair. Leave overnight, then comb through with a fine-toothed nit comb and rinse off. A drop of tea tree oil in hair conditioner two or three times a week is a very good preventive measure.

* Cockroaches, moths and rodents all hate sage, so tie bunches round the home.
* Burn some citronella candles to deter mosquitoes when you're sitting outside on a summer evening.
* Instead of mothballs, try using pieces of muslin that have been soaked in some cedarwood, camphor or lavender oil and placing them around the house, especially in wardrobes.
* If your cat or dog brings home fleas, vacuum the carpets and soft furnishings and wash what you can in boiling water. Spray tea tree and eucalyptus oils diluted in water onto the furniture and carpets, and don't forget to treat their bedding and baskets, too.
* Comb through the animal's coat with a mixture of olive oil, mint, eucalyptus and tea tree oil, squashing or drowning the fleas you comb out, then shampoo with a mild baby shampoo with a few drops of tea tree and eucalyptus mixed in.
* People with asthma associated with dust mite allergies should remove items such as wall-to-wall carpets and over-stuffed soft furnishings.
* To neutralize dust mites in these areas, just make a cup of very strong black tea, put it in a sprayer and then spray direct onto problem areas.
* To get rid of aphids (e.g. greenfly and blackfly), spider mites and scale mites, steep two garlic cloves in a litre of water for 24 hours; spray all over the affected plants.
* Is there an ants' nest in your garden? Instead of treating them with chemicals, pour a kettle of boiling

water over them. Pure lemon juice works as well, but it's better to save it for use in detox drinks and recipes.
● To keep wasps away from a picnic or any outdoor meal, all you need do is half-fill a tumbler with some fruit juice and then secure a paper lid over the top – you can hold it in place with a rubber band. Pierce a hole through the paper with a pencil. The wasps will crawl through, attracted by the scent of the juice, but will not be able to get out again.

THE AIR WE BREATHE

When you are in an area with a lot of traffic, you know all about it. The air even smells poisonous – and it is. Traffic emissions contain the following toxins:
● Benzene (which is linked to leukaemia)
● Carbon monoxide (makes you tired, causes memory

Cooking warnings
● Avoid non-stick pans coated in perfluorooctanioic acids (PFOAs), subsequently found in foods cooked in them.
● Avoid polyethylene terephthalate (PET) plastic containers for heating foods in a microwave or storing wet foods or acidic liquids, such as wine or juice.
● Avoid boil-in-the-bag foods, because of the risk of antimony leaking from the plastic. Smoking cooking oils or charred meats, e.g. on barbecues, can be carcinogenic to inhale and to eat, so don't have the heat too high.

Radon

Radon is a radioactive gas formed from the breakdown of uranium in the earth. It is more common in areas with a lot of granite and limestone in the topsoil. Breathing in tiny particles of radon can increase your chance of getting lung cancer, but there are measures that can reduce your risk level. Contact your environmental health officer, or look at the Health Protection Agency's website at: www.hpa.org.uk/radiation/radar/index.htm.

loss, can cause chest pain and miscarriage)
• Diesel particles (these have been linked to circulatory disease and lung cancer)
• Petrol (may damage the nervous system and lungs)
• Polycyclic aromatic hydrocarbons (linked to reproductive problems and cancer)
• Total petroleum hydrocarbons (may affect circulatory and immune systems, the skin, lungs and eyes).
You are breathing in even more of these chemicals while you are sitting in your car than out in the street, because the air pumped in for the heating and air conditioning systems is at ground level where the exhaust fumes are pumped out.

Rural life

Do you think that you would be better off moving to the country instead? Well, the air there can be full of agricultural pesticides and fertilizers. These contain:

- Carbamates (some experts think disrupt the nervous system and can cause rashes and fatigue at low levels)
- Organochlorines (thought to build up in fat cells and over the long term can cause weakness and tremors)
- Organophosphates (high levels are fatal and low levels are linked to skin rashes and fatigue)
- Pyrethroids (linked to nervous system damage and respiratory system irritation).

COMBATING THE PROBLEM

So what can you do, given that the average human needs to breathe between 8,000 and 10,000 litres of air a day to stay alive? Here are some useful suggestions to try:

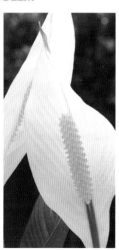

- You can open all the windows and try to ventilate your house as much as possible
- Houseplants can help to reduce the levels of formaldehyde, benzene and other contaminants in the atmosphere as they absorb them as a source of food. Palms,

bamboo and peace lilies are all good decontaminants
● Outdoors, try to choose routes that are tree-lined, or where there are a lot of plants, because the process of photosynthesis removes some harmful gases from the atmosphere and produces more oxygen
● Take particular care when exercising outdoors as you are breathing in huge lungfuls of air and your circulation is speeding it rapidly round your system
● Cyclists are advised to wear masks for riding in towns and in the countryside.

Look after your health

Don't panic! If you have a respiratory disease, such as asthma or emphysema, you might consider moving to a less polluted part of the country, although airborne toxins are pretty endemic and traces have even been found in tests on people who live on some of the UK's most remote islands.

Healthy guidelines

Concentrate on avoiding the toxins that you can do something about – in the products you buy. Read the labels carefully; if there is a long string of complex chemicals, give those products a miss. Choose natural ingredients, such as essential oils, herbs and sea salts, and look for certified organic brands. You can't avoid all the toxins in modern life, but if you try not to ingest them voluntarily, you will be taking a huge step towards looking after your health.

GLOSSARY

Acetaldehyde Toxic intermediary product which is created when alcohol is broken down by the liver.

Adrenaline Hormone released by adrenal gland in response to fear or stress.

Amino acids Building blocks of proteins needed to grow, repair cells and maintain muscles. Twelve essential amino acids are produced by body, but we need a further eight from our food.

Antibody Substance produced by white blood cells to attack and neutralize invaders, e.g. bacteria and viruses.

Antioxidants Chemical that helps neutralize free radicals and prevent damage to cells. Some occur naturally in the body; others supplied by betacarotene, vitamin C, vitamin E, etc.

Betacarotene Antioxidant converted in the intestine to retinol, which is essential for healthy skin and eyesight.

Carcinogen Substance capable of causing cancer.

Chelation Process in which chemical chelating agents are administered intravenously to combine with heavy metals in body and help neutralize them.

Cholesterol Fatty substance made by liver; used to form bile salts, hormones and other body cells; high levels in blood can build up in arteries and make them narrow.

Cortisol Stress hormone produced by adrenal gland.

Diuretic Substance that increases volume of urine passed.

Essential fatty acids (EFAs) Linoleic, linolenic and arachidonic acids are substances the body needs but doesn't produce (although it can make the other two from linoleic acid).

Food allergy Extreme immune system reaction to a food.

Food intolerance Adverse reaction to a food or ingredient in a food that can make you feel unwell.

Free radicals Unstable molecules with a negative electrical charge that cause cells to age and degenerate.

Glutathione Amino acid that enables liver to break down several kinds of toxins, including acetaldehyde.

Healing crisis Syndrome in which symptoms get worse before they get better; during a detox this could occur when stored toxins are released into the bloodstream.

Heavy metals Metallic elements we ingest through food, air and water that build up in the body tissues.

Hypothyroidism Syndrome in which thyroid gland does not produce enough essential hormones, causing fatigue, intolerance of cold, muscle weakness, slower heart rate.

Immune system Collective name for mechanisms by which body fights invaders, e.g. bacteria, viruses, toxic micro-organisms; plays role in control of cancerous cells and is responsible for allergies.

Lactoferrin Antibacterial agent found in sweat, saliva and mucous membranes in the respiratory system.

Lymphatic system System of vessels in which lymph fluid is drained from body tissues and white blood cells are directed to areas where they are required to fight invaders.

Parabens Preservatives used in cosmetics and personal care products such as deodorants.

Phthalate Substance added to plastics to make them more flexible, and a solvent used in several cosmetic products.

Phytonutrients Nutrients that come from plants.

Placebo Chemically inert substance given to a control group during drug tests; it can have a positive effect simply because patient believes it will.

Probiotics Beneficial micro-organisms in digestive tract and help protect it from bacteria, yeasts and viruses.

Volatile organic compounds (VOCs) Substances used widely in paint, paint strippers, petrol, aerosol sprays, dry-cleaning fluid and many other common household products.

USEFUL INFORMATION

Action on Smoking and Health (ASH)
102 Clifton Street,
London EC2A 4HW
Tel: 0800 169 0169
www.ash.org.uk

Alcoholics Anonymous
PO Box 1
Stonebow House, Stonebow,
York YO1 7NJ
Tel: 0845 769 7555
www.alcoholics-
anonymous.org.uk

Allergy UK
3 White Oak Square,
London Road, Swanley,
Kent BR8 7AG
Helpline 01322 619898
www.allergyuk.org

Aromatherapy Consortium
PO Box 6522
Desborough,Kettering,
Northants NN14 2YX
Tel: 0870 7743477
www.aromatherapy-
regulation.co.uk

Asthma UK
Summit House,
70 Wilson Street,
London EC2A 2DB
Tel: 020 7786 5000
www.asthma.org.uk

British Association for Counselling and Psychotherapy
BACP House,
35–37 Albert Street, Rugby,
Warwickshire CV21 2SG
Tel: 0870 443 5252
www.bacp.co.uk

British Heart Foundation
14 Fitzhardinge Street,
London W1H 6DH
Tel: 020 7935 0185
www.bhf.org.uk

British Nutrition Foundation
High Holborn House,
52–54 High Holborn,
London WC1V 6RQ
Tel: 020 7404 6504
www.nutrition.org.uk

Cancer Research UK
PO Box 123
Lincoln's Inn Fields,
London Wc2A 3PX
Tel: 020 7242 0200
www.cancerresearchuk.org

National Institute of Medical Herbalists
Elm House,
54 Mary Arches Street,
Exeter EX4 3BA
Tel: 01392 426022
www.nimh.org.uk

Friends of the Earth
26–28 Underwood Street,
London N1 7JQ
Tel: 020 7490 1555
www.foe.co.uk

General Osteopathic Council
176 Tower Bridge Road,
London SE1 3LU
Tel: 020 7357 6655
www.osteopathy.org.uk

Narcotics Anonymous
202 City Road,
London EC1V 2PH
Tel: 0845 3733366
www.ukna.org

College of Naturopathic Medicine UK
Unit 1, Bulrushes Farm,
Coombe Hill Road,
East Grinstead,
West Sussex RH19 4LZ
Tel: 01342 410 505
www.naturopathy-uk.com

Soil Association
Bristol House, 40–56 Victoria
Street, Bristol, BS1 6BY
Tel: 0117 314 5000
www.soilassociation.org

The Transcendental Meditation Association
Beacon House, Willow Walk,
Skelmersdale, Lancs
Tel: 0870 5143733
www.t-m.org.uk

The Vipassana Trust
Vipassana Centre Dhamma,
Dipa, Harewood End
Herefordshire HR2 8JS
Tel: 01989 730234
www.dhamma.org

Useful websites

www.chem-tox.com
(research on the effects of
chemicals and pesticides)

www.foodnews.org/tools.php
(pesticides used on fruit and
vegetables)

www.dwi.gov.uk
(Drinking Water Inspectorate)

www.kombuchatea.co.uk
(for advice on water filters)

**www.andalucia.com/health
/alternative-health**
(descriptions of therapies)

www.thewellnessstore.co.uk
(for supplements, natural
health and beauty)

www.highernature.co.uk
(supplements)

www.healthydirect.co.uk
(supplements)

**www.nealsyardremedies.
com**
(natural health and beauty)

http://flowervr.com/
(flower remedies)

www.detoku.com
(foot patches)

www.natureswisdom.co.uk
(flower and light essences)

www.greenpeople.co.uk
(natural personal care)

www.SoOrganic.co.uk
(organic shopping)

www.gogreen.cellande.co.uk
(a green directory)

www.spiritofnature.co.uk
(natural products, from
clothes to cosmetics)

**www.theremustbeabetter
way.co.uk**
(products for allergy
sufferers)

www.botanicals.co.uk
(hair care)

**www.honestycosmetics.
co.uk**
(as the name implies)

www.ecomerchant.co.uk
(sustainable building
materials)

www.planetnatural.com
(organic gardening)

www.gaias-garden.co.uk/tips
(natural advice)

**www.organicgardening.
co.uk**

www.ecopaints.co.uk

www.ieko.co.uk
(natural paints)

www.earthbornpaints.co.uk

**www.greenbuildingstore.
co.uk**

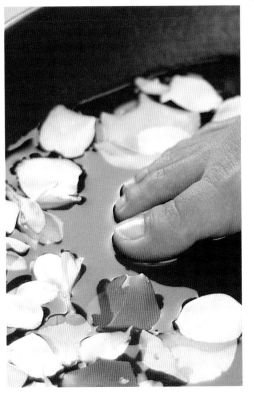

FURTHER READING

General nutrition

Brewer, Sarah, *Encyclopedia of Vitamins, Minerals and Herbal Supplements* (Robinson)

Carper, Jean, *The Food Pharmacy* (Pocket Books)

Clarke, Jane, *Bodyfoods for Busy People* (Quadrille)

Lawrence, Felicity, *Not on the Label: What Really Goes into the Food on your Plate* (Penguin)

McKeith, Gillian, *You are What You Eat* (Michael Joseph)

Ursell, Amanda, *What are you Really Eating?* (Hay House)

Giving up bad habits

Carr, Allen, *Allen Carr's Easy Way to Stop Smoking* (Penguin)

Paul, Gill, *Collins Gem Stop Smoking* (HarperCollins)

Pluymen, Bert, *The Thinking Person's Guide to Sobriety* (Griffin)

The Easy Way to Control Alcohol (Arcturus Foulsham)

Detox guides

Gittleman, Ann Louise, *The Fast Track Detox Diet* (Century)

Dr Joshi's Holistic Detox (Hodder)

Kenton, Leslie, *The New Raw Energy* (Vermilion)

Kenton, Leslie, *Power Juices* (Vermilion)

Scrivner, Jane, *Detox Yourself* (Piatkus)

Scrivner, Jane, *La Stone Therapy Manual* (Piatkus)

Scrivner, Jane, *Total Detox: 6 Ways to Revitalise Your Life* (Piatkus)

Vorderman, Carol, *Carol Vorderman's Detox Recipes* (Virgin)

Vorderman, Carol, *Carol Vorderman's 30-day Cellulite Plan* (Virgin)

Vorderman, Carol, *Detox for Life* (Virgin)

Williams, Xandria, *The Liver Detox Plan* (Vermilion)

Detox: How to Cleanse and Revitalise your Body, your Home and your Life (Rodale)

Emotional health

Berne, Eric, *Games People Play* (Penguin)

Bodhipaksa, *Guided Meditations for Calmness, Awareness and Love* (Wisdom Books)

Cameron, Julia, *Artist's Way* (Jeremy P. Tarcher)

Chopra, Deepak, *The Seven Spiritual Laws of Success* (Excel Books)

Golman, Daniel P., *Emotional Intelligence* (Bantam)

Harrison, Eric, *Teach Yourself to Meditate* (Piatkus)

Kornfield, Jack, *After the Ecstasy, the Laundry* (Bantam)

Kornfield, Jack, *Meditation for Beginners* (Bantam)

Organic living

Hollender, Jeffrey, *Naturally Clean* (New Society)

Palmer, Sue, *Toxic Childhood* (Orion)

Perry, Luddene, and Schultz, Dan, *A Field Guide to Buying Organic* (Bantam)

Sandbeck, Ellen, *Organic Housekeeping* (Scribner)

Soil Association, *The Really Good Life* (Cassell)

Sullivan, Karen, *A Healthy House – Naturally*

Trask, Crissy, *It's Easy Being Green* (Gibbs Smith)

INDEX

Look out for further titles in the Collins Gem series.

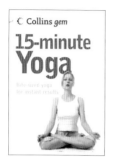

Collins *gem*

15-minute Yoga

Bite-sized yoga for instant results

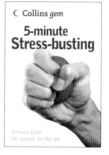

Collins *gem*

5-minute Stress-busting

Instant calm for people on the go

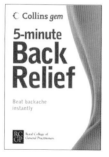

Collins *gem*

5-minute Back Relief

Beat backache instantly

Royal College of General Practitioners

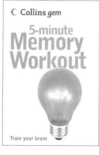

Collins *gem*

5-minute Memory Workout

Train your brain